Basics of Nutrition
Macronutrients & Micronutrients

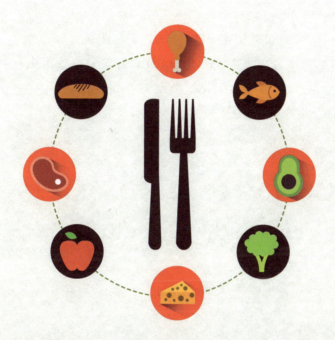

Explains the food nutrition basics

Dr. SU LI, Ph.D.

https://www.tiktok.com/@e.nutrition

**Basics of Nutrition
Macronutrients & Micronutrients**

This book explains the basics of food nutrition.
You will learn the macronutrients (carbohydrates, protein, water, and fat) and micronutrients (vitamins and minerals) needed in our daily eating patterns for good health and wellness.
With easily understandable and facts-based content supported by informative graphics, this book gives you the knowledge and confidence to assess and enhance your approach to nutrition.

Basics of Nutrition

Macronutrients and Micronutrients

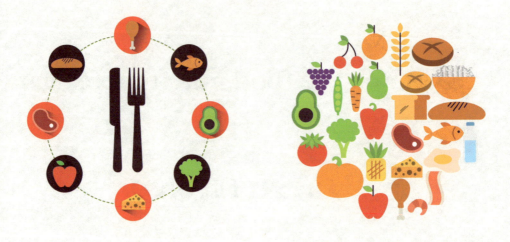

https://www.tiktok.com/@e.nutrition

Basics of Nutrition

Macronutrients & Micronutrients

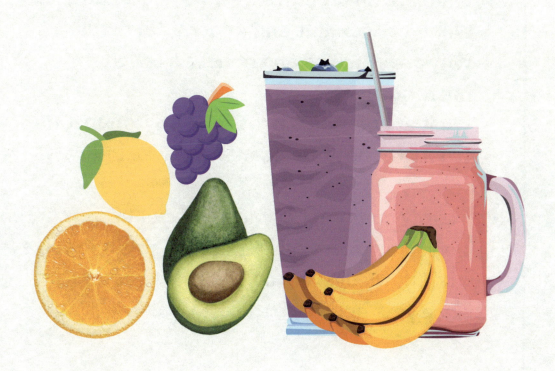

SU LI

Basics of Nutrition

This book explains the basics of nutrition we get from food. You will learn the nutrition needed in our daily eating pattern for health and wellness.

- **You will get to know the macronutrients, including water, protein, fat, and carbohydrates.**
- What are macronutrients and micronutrients?
- What are vitamins and minerals in foods?
- Why are vitamins and minerals called micronutrients?
- What are phytonutrients and phytonutrition?
- What are the antioxidants and free radicals?

With easily comprehensible and facts-based content supported by informative graphics, this book gives you the knowledge and confidence to assess and enhance your approach to nutrition.

https://www.tiktok.com/@e.nutrition

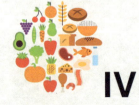

Preface

Basics of Nutrition: Macronutrients and Micronutrients

The rise in awareness of healthy lifestyles worldwide is escalating the growth of the wellness supplements market.

Our belief is that everyone is empowered to embrace a healthy lifestyle through the food we enjoy and the life we lead.

Our bodies are as unique as our personalities, so we strive to find an optimized eating pattern that works for us individually.

This book gives you the basics of nutrition, from what they are in nature and what they do in our bodies. The nutrition facts are explained with informative graphics, making it easy to understand.

This book will give you a clear picture of macronutrients and micronutrients and enable you to make informed choices that are best suited to you about what, when, and how to eat responsibly for health, wellness, and happiness.

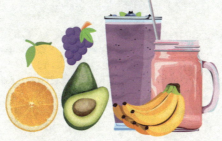

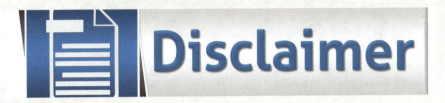

Disclaimer

This book is intended to provide broad guidance only and is not a substitute for professional medical advice, diagnosis, or treatment. If you have any concerns about your medical issues, dietary needs, or your interest in, questions about, or usage of dietary supplements, or what could possibly be best for your overall wellness, you must always seek the opinion of your physician or fellow licensed healthcare expert.

Never disregard or delay seeking professional medical advice based on a concept you read in this book, our e-books and books, our websites, our videos and audios, articles or social media.

The author and publisher of this book are not medical professionals, and the information provided throughout is based on research, personal experience, and general health and wellness information and expertise. While every effort has been made to ensure the precision and accuracy of the information provided, the author and publisher render no implicit or explicit representations or assurances concerning the content contained in this book's completeness, accuracy, reliability, suitability, or availability for any purpose.

The reader acknowledges full responsibility for any actions taken in reliance on the information in this book. The author and publisher bear no responsibility for any direct, indirect, consequential, or incidental damages resulting from the use or inability to use the material in this book.

Before undertaking any new health or wellness program, making dietary changes, or commencing a new exercise regimen, it is critical to consult a licensed healthcare expert. Individual results may vary, and no assurances are offered concerning the outcomes or effects of following the advice or suggestions in this book.

The information provided in this book should not substitute any medical advice. Any reference to third-party websites or resources is provided for convenience only and does not indicate endorsement of the material, perspectives, or services offered by other websites.

By reading this book, you consent that you have carefully reviewed this disclaimer, and you agree to utilize the knowledge contained therein at your own discretion. Always prioritize your health and well-being by seeking tailored counsel and direction from a certified healthcare practitioner.

SuTasty Inc. owns and regulates all content copyright, and any replication of this company's content without permission is prohibited.

Table of Contents

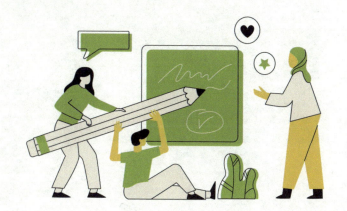

02 ### Nutrients
Six groups of nutrients, Macronutrients, and Micronutrients

06 ### Disclaimer

20 ### Water | the Macronutrient
Water, the vital nutrient.

27 ### Carbohydrates
The primary energy source for the human body. Monosaccharides, disaccharides, starch, and fiber. Glycemic Index (GI), Glycemic Load (GL), Empty calories, Sugar Substitutes (saccharin, sucralose, stevia)

75 ### Fats
Unsaturated saturated fat, Essential fatty acids (ALA, LA), DHA and EPA, cholesterol.

87 ### Proteins
Nine essential amino acids, complete protein, complementary proteins, protein in the body, enzymes, hormones, collagen

Table of Contents

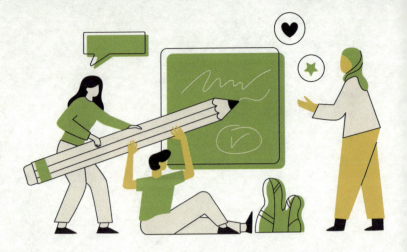

110 **Phytochemicals and Phytonutrients**
Carotenoids, flavonoids, indoles, allicin; the rainbow color of foods

122 **What happens when we eat?**
Digestion, metabolism, balanced diet

130 **Antioxidants and free radicals**
Natural antioxidants from foods, the role of antioxidants, oxidative stress and free radicals, phytonutrients and antioxidants

136 **Units of Measurement**

141 **Index**

142 **About the author**

Introduction

Explains the basics of nutrition

This book explains the basics of the macronutrients and micronutrients required by our bodies to stay healthy. This book also explained the basics of phytonutrients and natural antioxidants from foods that may benefit our health.

In this book, we explained the nutrients and illustrated what they are and what they do in our bodies. We explained carbohydrates, proteins, fats, and water, collectively called macronutrients. In addition, we also briefly presented the micronutrients, vitamins, and minerals. Our two other books explicitly explain vitamins and minerals in this book series: Basics of Vitamins & Basics of MInerals.

For more information and fun facts about macronutrients, vitamins, and minerals, please follow us on our TikTok and YouTube channels, where videos explain food nutrition in a fun and easy-understandable way.

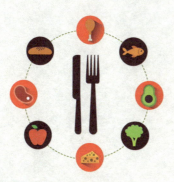
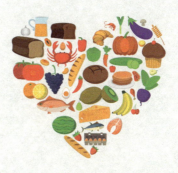

What are nutrition, nutrients, and diet?

Diet and nutrition are fundamental in maintaining our health.

What is nutrition?
Nutrition is a human process of utilizing food for the growth, metabolism, and repair of tissues. Nutrition provides the body with the nutrients necessary for good health. Essentially, nutrition is the nourishment of the body via the foods we eat.

Eating nutritiously enables us to enjoy the well-being that comes with good health. Adequate nutrition is vital for our body and mind to be healthy and well-maintained, have the best chance at fighting disease, and operate functionally well.

What are nutrients?
Nutrients are the nourishing substances in food that give us energy, allow our bodies to grow, and keep us feeling healthy. Water is a unique type of nutrient, giving us hydration. The nutrients in our food are categorized into macronutrients and micronutrients.

What is diet?
Diet refers to the total amount of food consumed by individuals.
Diet is the foods and beverages we usually eat and drink; diet is also called eating pattern.

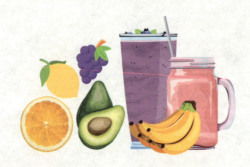

Macronutrients and Micronutrients

We get our nourishment mostly from macronutrients, the primary dietary players, but micronutrients are no less essential. A balanced diet contains many different types of both.

Based on the amount required by the human body for normal metabolism, growth, and physical well-being, nutrients are divided into two categories: macronutrients consisting of water, proteins, carbohydrates, and fats, and micronutrients comprised of vitamins and minerals.

Fats are the most energy-dense macronutrient, whereas carbohydrates are quantitatively the most essential dietary energy source for most populations.

Proteins are vital structural and functional components within every body cell and are essential for our growth, repair, and health maintenance.

Minerals and vitamins, found in small amounts in most foods, are essential for our normal metabolic function. This book focuses on minerals; the other two books in this series (Basics of Nutrition) will separately focus on vitamins and macronutrients. Now, let's start our journey of minerals, and you will be well-informed mineral-wise when you design your diet to stay healthier and happier.

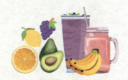

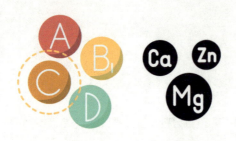 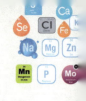

Vitamins and Minerals
(A Brief introduction)

Vitamins and minerals are essential substances that our bodies need to function normally. Several minerals are necessary for health, including sodium, chloride, potassium, calcium, phosphorus, magnesium, sulfur, iron, zinc, copper, selenium, iodine, cobalt, fluoride, manganese, and molybdenum.

The known vitamins are vitamin C, vitamins A, D, E, and K, choline (B vitamin complex), and the B vitamins: thiamin, riboflavin, niacin, pantothenic acid, vitamin B6, vitamin B12, biotin, and folate.

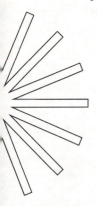

Unique nutritional needs

There is no one-size-fits-all in nutrition.
Your optimal intake of each macronutrient and micronutrient depends on numerous factors. Your age, gender, genetics, metabolism, level of physical activity, and personal preferences all have a part to play in establishing the best foods to keep working optimally.

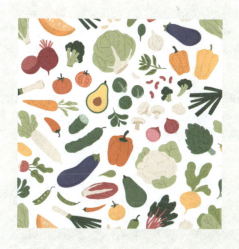

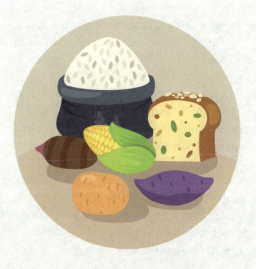

Veggies
Veggies are full of micronutrients and flavor, providing variety and nourishment.

Carbs
Carbohydrates are a major energy source for the body and provide fiber for healthy digestion.

Disclaimer

This book is intended to provide broad guidance only and is not a substitute for professional medical advice, diagnosis, or treatment. If you have any concerns about your medical issues, dietary needs, or your interest in, questions about, or usage of dietary supplements, or what could be best for your overall wellness, you must always seek the opinion of your physician or fellow licensed healthcare expert.

Never disregard or delay seeking professional medical advice based on a concept you read in this book, e-book, on our website, video and audio, articles, or social media.

The author and publisher of this book are not medical professionals, and the information provided throughout is based on research, personal experience, and general health and wellness information and expertise. While every effort has been made to ensure the precision and accuracy of the information provided, the author and publisher render no implicit or explicit representations or assurances concerning the content contained in this book's completeness, accuracy, reliability, suitability, or availability for any purpose.

The reader acknowledges full responsibility for any actions taken in reliance on the information in this book. The author and publisher bear no responsibility for any direct, indirect, consequential, or incidental damages resulting from the use or inability to use the material in this book.

Before undertaking any new health or wellness program, making dietary changes, or commencing a new exercise regimen, it is critical to consult a licensed healthcare expert. Individual results may vary, and no assurances are offered concerning the outcomes or effects of following the advice or suggestions in this book.

The information provided in this book should not substitute any medical advice. Any reference to third-party websites or resources is provided for convenience only and does not indicate endorsement of the material, perspectives, or services offered by other websites.

By reading this book, you consent that you have carefully reviewed this disclaimer, and agree to utilize the knowledge contained therein at your discretion. Always prioritize your health and well-being by seeking tailored counsel and direction from a certified healthcare practitioner.

SuTasty Inc. owns and regulates all content copyright, and any replication of this channel's content without permission is prohibited.

Nutrients
The six groups of nutrients

What are nutrients?

Nutrients are the nourishing substances in food that provide water, energy, or calories, promote the growth and maintenance of the human body, and regulate body processes. In other words, nutrients are the nourishing substances in food that give us water, energy, and building materials, allow our body to grow and develop, maintain the health of our body, and keep us feeling healthy.

six groups of nutrients		
carbohydrate	protein	minerals
vitamins	fat	water

The six groups of nutrients

Nutrients provide water and energy, promote growth, development, and maintenance of the body, and regulate body processes.

The nutrients help regulate numerous processes in our body, for example, the heart-beating and the digestion of food in the stomach. Nutrients include carbohydrates, fats, protein, water, minerals, and vitamins. The nutrients are grouped into six main groups:

1. Carbohydrates.
2. Fats.
3. Protein.
4. Vitamins
5. Minerals
6. Water.

The six groups of nutrients are further divided into two major categories: macronutrients and micronutrients.

Most foods provide a mix of nutrients. For example, a cake gives carbohydrates and fats, but it also gives you some vitamins and minerals depending on the cake's ingredients. Food contains more than just nutrients; it may include flavouring, colouring, caffeine, phytonutrients, and other substances.

The macronutrients and micronutrients

What are macronutrients?
Macronutrients are water, carbohydrates, protein, and fats. Macro means large. The body needs large amounts of water, carbohydrates, fats, and protein, so they are named macronutrients. Carbohydrates, fats, and proteins are also called energy-yielding nutrients. Energy-yielding nutrients are the nutrients that can be burned as fuel to provide energy for the body. Carbohydrates, fats, and protein can be burned to give kilocalories; therefore, they are energy-yielding nutrients.

Macronutrients

| Carbohydrate | Protein | Fat | Water |

Energy-yielding nutrients

| Carbohydrate | Protein | Fat |

The six groups of nutrients

Carbohydrates: Carbohydrates are the body's primary energy source. Carbohydrates are a large class of nutrients, including starches, fibers, and sugar.	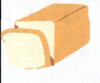
Fats Fats are also called lipids. Fats are a group of fatty substances, including triglycerides and cholesterol, that are not soluble in water and produce rich energy sources and structural-building substances in the body's cells.	
Proteins Proteins are a group of nutrients that are the major structural part of the body's cells and are found in large quantities in animal foods.	
Vitamins and Minerals Vitamins and Minerals provide no calories. They are found in a variety of foods, especially fruits and vegetables. Vitamins and minerals are essential in small amounts to maintain the body, regulate body processes, and allow for the body's growth and reproduction.	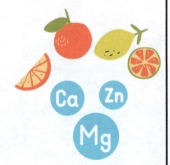
Water Water is the most vital nutrient that plays a role in all bodily processes and makes up just over half of the body weight.	

Macronutrients and Micronutrients

The six groups of nutrients can be further classified into two major categories: macronutrients and micronutrients.

Macronutrients are the nutrients we need in large amounts daily.

Carbohydrates, fat, and protein are the macronutrients that provide the human body with calories or energy; therefore, they are also referred to as energy-yielding nutrients.

Equally important, water is a macronutrient. Water is a vital macronutrient. Our bodies need water to stay healthy, and about 60% of our body weight is water. Water does not provide calories to the body. However, water is a crucial nutrient for all body cells and tissues to function properly. We will talk about water in further detail in the following chapters.

Micronutrients are vitamins and minerals. Our bodies require vitamins and minerals in small amounts.

Macronutrients			
Water	Carbs	Protein	Minerals
Micronutrients			
Vitamins		Minerals	

Carbohydrates | the Macronutrient

Carbohydrates are a large class of nutrients, including sugars, starch, and fibres. Carbohydrates function as the body's primary source of energy.

We will talk about sugar, starch, and fibres. We will discuss the common sugars we usually see and use: sucrose (table sugar or white sugar), glucose, lactose, fructose, and maltose. The natural sugar in fruits is fructose, and the natural sugar in milk is lactose. Table sugar or white sugar is sucrose, which is sold in grocery stores and added to foods.

Then, we will talk about starch and fibres, which are also sugar in nature but polysaccharides, meaning that in each of their molecules, hundreds and thousands of glucose are linked together.

Carbohydrates are the primary energy source for our bodies. Our bodies break down the carbohydrates we eat and digest carbs into glucose, and glucose, or blood sugar, is the primary energy source for your body's cells, tissues, and organs.

Carbohydrate		
Sugar	Starch	Fiber

Protein | the Macronutrient

Protein is a nutrient that is a significant part of the body's cells. From our hair to the toe, We have proteins in us.

Protein is made of amino acids assembled in chains; protein performs many bodily functions. Protein is part of every cell, tissue, and organ.

Proteins perform both structural and functional roles in our bodies. Besides its role as an essential part of cells, protein can be burned to provide energy, although the body prefers to burn carbohydrates and fat, so protein can be used to build new cells.

Good protein sources from animal-based foods are beef, meat, poultry, eggs, milk, and cheese.
Plant-based foods such as grains, beans, vegetables, potatoes, and sweet potatoes contain protein but in smaller quantities than meat.

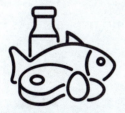 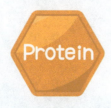 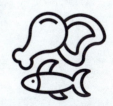

Proteins

Fat | the Macronutrient

Fat is a macronutrient found in many foods. Consuming fats is vital to the body's function, including processes such as hormone production, brain activity, and the body's absorption of other nutrients from the diet.

Fats provide a rich source of energy to cells. Fat is a nutrient that supplies a rich energy source to the body. We should aim to get one-third of our calories from fat.

Butter, margarine, vegetable oils, and mayonnaise contain fats. Fat is also present in many foods and makes foods tasty. Fatty steaks in meat have fats, and you can find fat under the skin of poultry. There is also fat in milk and cheese except for fat-free milk and dairy products. Fats are also contained in baked goods such as cakes, fried foods, nuts, and other foods.

Fats, protein, and carbohydrates are energy-yielding nutrients that provide us with calories. Most of the calories we eat come from carbohydrates and fats. Only about 15% of total calories come from protein, depending on individual diets people have.

Fats we eat are broken down into triglycerides that travel in the blood to wherever they will be used or stored. Naturally, Most foods contain different types of fats: saturated and unsaturated fats (monosaturated and polyunsaturated fats).

Fats

Micronutrients: vitamins and minerals.

Micronutrients are vitamins and minerals. Micro means small. The body needs vitamins and minerals in small amounts, so these two types of nutrients are called micronutrients. Although Vitamins and minerals are the nutrients required by the body in small quantities, these play significant roles in the body's vital functions.

In summary, the macronutrients needed by the body are water, carbohydrates, fats, and protein. In comparison, the micronutrients are minerals and vitamins, which our body needs in small amounts.

Micronutrients	
Vitamins	Minerals

Vitamins | Micronutrients

Vitamins are organic compounds made by plants or animals. Vitamins are noncaloric organic nutrients in various foods essential in small quantities to regulate body processes, maintain the body, and allow growth and reproduction.

Vitamins and minerals, along with water, are zero-calorie-generating nutrients. They do not provide calories but are vital for humans to stay healthy.

Vitamins are nutrients we need to obtain from our foods to ensure optimal health and prevent nutritional deficiencies. Aim to include various veggies and fruits in your diet to pack all the necessary vitamins.

Food has 13 different vitamins and one vitaminB-complex choline. They are Vitamin A, Vitamin D, Vitamin E, Vitamin K, vitamin C, vitamin B1 (thiamin), vitamin B2 (riboflavin), vitamin B3 (niacin), vitamin B5 (pantothenic acid), vitamin B6, vitamin B7 (biotin), vitamin B9 (folate), vitamin B12(cobalamin).

B vitamins are essential in keeping the nervous system healthy and helping our bodies release energy from the foods we eat. Folate helps with brain and spinal cord development in unborn babies.

Vitamins are essential in small quantities to regulate body processes and maintain the body and all growth and reproduction. Vitamins assist in the processes of the body that keep us healthy. For example, vitamin A is needed by the eyes for vision in dim light.

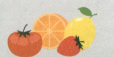

Vitamins | Micronutrients

Vitamin C helps maintain healthy skin, blood vessels, and cartilage and plays a role in collagen production, which keeps skin elasticity and strength. Vitamin C is also an antioxidant that protects cells and tissues from oxidative damage and contributes to healing from colds and flu.

Vitamins A and E are potent antioxidants, helping protect cells from free radicals and aging. Vitamin A contributes to cell renewal and repair. Vitamin E reduces the effects of skin aging and the risk of skin cancer. Sources of vitamin A include carrots, sweet potatoes, and some types of fish, such as herring and salmon.

Vitamin D is unique because it is a hormone we can make in our bodies with sunlight exposure. Dietary sources include egg yolks, oily fish, and fortified foods.

Vitamin K is essential for wound healing and blood clotting. Sources include green leafy vegetables and vegetable oils.

Vitamins are found in many foods, including fruits, vegetables, grains, meat, poultry, dairy products, and other foods.

Micronutrients	
Vitamins	Minerals

Minerals | the Micronutrients

Our bodies need certain minerals to function well. A variety of foods contain both vitamins and minerals. So, a varied diet will help you meet your mineral requirements.

Minerals are inorganic chemical elements from soil, rock, or water. Minerals are absorbed from the environment by plants as they grow and by animals that eat these plants. There are many minerals, each with healthful benefits. We should include each type in our diet regularly. Our bodies require minerals in relatively more significant quantities, such as calcium, chloride, magnesium, phosphorous, potassium, sulfur, and sodium. Other minerals, iron, copper, zinc, selenium, iodine, fluoride, manganese, molybdenum, and cobalt are needed in trace quantities. Calcium is a vital component of bone and teeth and an essential nutrient for the nervous system, muscles, and heart. Sources of calcium include milk, yogurt, spinach, and many more.

Iodine is essential for normal thyroid function and the production of thyroid hormones, which are involved in many processes in the body, such as growth, brain development, and bone maintenance. Thyroid hormones also regulate the metabolism. Sources of iodine include fish, iodized table salt, eggs, seaweed, and dairy products.

Iron is an essential mineral required for the body's growth and development. Iron is needed for the body to make the proteins hemoglobin and myoglobin. Hemoglobin is the protein in red blood cells carrying oxygen from the lungs to all body parts; Myoglobin is the protein that provides oxygen to muscles. Iron is also required by the body to make some hormones. Iron may also have other benefits, such as improving immune and brain functions. Sources of iron include seafood, meat, poultry, Iron-fortified breakfast cereals and bread, beans and peas, nuts and seeds.

Minerals | the Micronutrients

Magnesium plays a role in more than 300 cellular processes, including energy production, nervous system function, and muscle contraction. Sources include avocados, nuts, and leafy greens.

Manganese helps make and activate some of the enzymes in the body that carry out biochemical reactions, such as breaking down foods. Sources include bread, nuts, and green vegetables.

Potassium is essential for blood pressure control, fluid balance, and muscle and nerve function. Sources include bananas, spinach, potatoes, and apricots.

Phosphorus helps the body build strong bones and also releases energy from food. Sources include meat, fish, dairy, poultry, oats and bread.

Selenium helps the immune system work efficiently, prevents damage to cells and tissues, and promotes the health of the reproductive systems. Sources of selenium include Brazil nuts, eggs, fish, and meat.

Zinc supports the immune system, hormone production, and fertility. Zinc can help reduce skin inflammation, support sound healing, and protect against sun damage. Sources include shellfish, meat, eggs, and chickpeas.

Micronutrients

Vitamins | Minerals

Water | the Macronutrient

Water is essential to life.
Water is vital in all bodily processes, making up just over half of the body's weight. Water supplies the medium where various body chemical changes occur, aiding digestion, absorption, circulation, and lubrication of body joints and soft tissues. As a major component of blood, water helps deliver nutrients to body cells and removes waste to the kidneys for excretion.

Many people have said, "You are what you eat."
The nutrients you eat can be found in your body.
As mentioned, water is the most plentiful nutrient in the body, accounting for about 50%-60% of your weight. Protein accounts for about 15% of your weight, fat for 15% to 25%, and carbohydrates for only 0.5%. The remainder of your weight includes minerals and traces of vitamins.

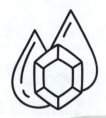 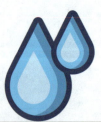 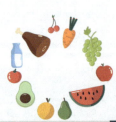 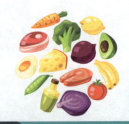

Water | the Macronutrient

Water, the macronutrient

Water is the main component of our body fluids and makes up more than half of our body weight. The body needs more water than any other nutrient, and we replenish it through the food we eat and what we drink. Water serves as a carrier. It distributes nutrients to cells and removes wastes through urine. It regulates body temperature and the electrolyte balance of our blood. Water is also essential for the body's metabolism.

Water is frequently classified as a macronutrient and shows on the USDA's list of macronutrients. This is because water needs to be consumed in (relatively) large quantities to survive. However, unlike protein, fat, and carbohydrates, water does not provide energy and therefore has zero calories.

Reference (water, the 4th macronutrient): https://www.nal.usda.gov/human-nutrition-and-food-safety/food-composition/macronutrients

Water – the Vital Nutrient

Water is a vital nutrient for us. The cells in our bodies are full of water. Almost all body cells need and depend on water to perform their functions. Water serves as the medium for chemical reactions required by the human body to stay alive. Water carries nutrients to the cells and carries away waste materials to the kidneys and out of the body, mainly in the urine.

Water is a vital nutrient for the human body for the following functions:

- Water maintains the health and integrity of every cell in the body. Water carries nutrients and oxygen to cells. Water is required to convert food eaten into energy in cells.
- The digestive secretions' water softens, dilutes, and liquefies the food to make digestion easier. Water also helps move food along the gastrointestinal tract. In addition, the difference in the fluid concentration on the two sides of the intestinal wall improves the absorption of nutrients.
- Water is the most abundant component of blood. Around 92% of blood is water, which maintains blood volume in the human body. So, Water keeps the bloodstream liquid enough to flow through blood vessels.

 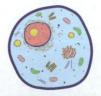

Water – the vital nutrient

- **Water regulates body temperature through sweating. Water in the blood also helps maintain average body temperature. For example, muscles work hard when people exercise and produce heat and energy. The body needs to eliminate the heat; blood goes to the muscles, picks up the heat, and circulates it to the skin. By sweating, the heat can be removed with some loss of water. The result is that the body cools down.**

- **Water also serves as an essential part of body cushion and body lubricants, helping to cushion the joints and internal organs and keeping tissues in the eyes, lungs, respiratory system, and air passages moist. In addition, water moistens mucous membranes (such as the lungs and mouth).**

- **Water helps eliminate the by-products of the body's metabolism, excess electrolytes (for example, sodium and potassium), and urea, a waste product formed through the processing of dietary protein.**

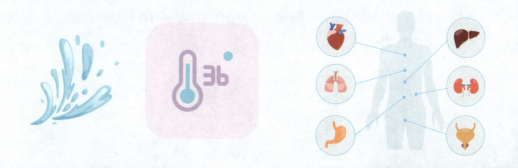

How much water do we need?

- Water is the most abundant substance that composes our bodies. About 50%-60% of an adult's body weight is water.

- You lose water daily through your breath, sweat, urine, and bowel movements. Therefore, for your body to function correctly, you must replenish its water supply by consuming water.

- The adequate intake for total water is based on how much fluid needs to be taken by adequately hydrated people each day. The amount required varies depending on factors such as age, weight, size, diet, activity, and the humidity and temperature of the environment.

- The Food and Nutrition Board of the INSTITUTE OF MEDICINE OF THE NATIONAL ACADEMIES determined that an adequate daily fluid intake is: for adult men 19 to 50 years old, the adequate daily intake (AI) of water is 3.7 liters. For adult women 19-50 years old, the AI is 2.7 liters daily. These recommendations cover fluids from water, other beverages, and food. About 20% of daily fluid intake usually comes from food, and the rest from drinks.

 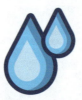

A healthy body maintains water at a constant level.

- The human body gets rid of the water it does not need through the kidneys and the skin. In addition, water is removed from the lungs and gastrointestinal tract to a lesser degree.
- Water is excreted as urine by the kidneys. In addition to urine, air released from the lungs contains water, and evaporation on the skin includes water. Water is essential to most bodily functions. However, the body cannot store water and needs fresh supplies daily.

References:
https://nap.nationalacademies.org/read/10925/chapter/6
National Academies of Sciences, Engineering, and Medicine. 2005. Dietary Reference Intakes for Water, Potassium, Sodium, Chloride, and Sulfate. Washington, DC: The National Academies Press. https://doi.org/10.17226/10925.

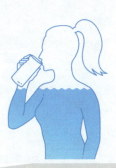

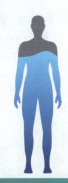

What does water do for you?

Required by the brain to produce hormones and neurotransmitters

Water forms saliva and digestive secretions

Water is required by body cells to perform their functions

Water required to convert food into energy in cells

Water acts a shock absorber for the brain and spinal cord

Helps deliver oxygen all over the body

Water is the major component of most body parts

Regulates body temperature through sweating and respiration

Water carries nutrients to body cells

Keeps mucosal membranes moist

lubricates joints

Flushes body waste mainly in urine

Water maintains blood volume

Water helps body cushion and body lubricants

Allows the body's cells to grow, reproduce, and survive

Keeps tissues in the eyes, lungs, and respiratory system and air passages moist

Carbohydrates

The primary energy source for the human body

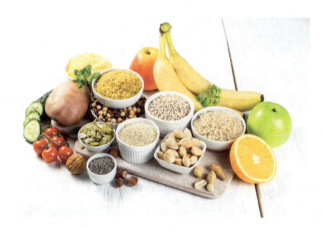

Carbohydrates are a large class of nutrients, including sugars, starches, and fibers, that function as the body's primary energy source.

Carbohydrates

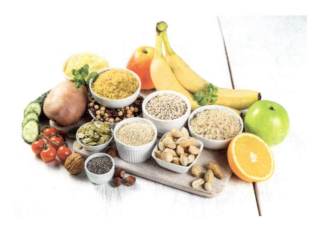

Sugars, starches, and fibers all belong to carbohydrates. Carbohydrates are the energy-yielding nutrient. All carbohydrates are made of the same three elements: carbon, hydrogen, and oxygen.

Grains, like oats and rice, are rich in carbohydrates. When grains such as wheat are ground, it produces flour to bake bread, tortillas, crackers, cookies, and cakes.

Carbohydrate is the primary energy source for most of us. Carbohydrates produce energy for our bodies, and carbohydrates can spare protein for the body's use. Carbohydrates can also assist in lipid/fat metabolism.

Carbohydrates

In this chapter, we talk about sugars, starch, and fibers.

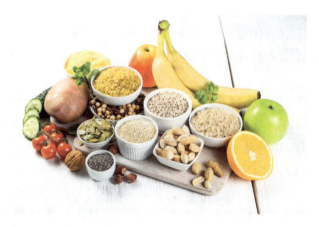

Sugars

Sugars are carbohydrates. The natural sugar in fruits is glucose and fructose, and the natural sugar in milk is lactose. Table sugar or cane sugar is added to foods and sold in grocery stores; table sugar is sucrose.

In this sugar section, we will talk about sugars including glucose, sucrose, fructose and lactose.

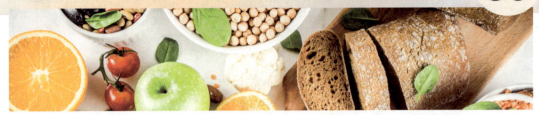

Simple carbohydrates and complex carbohydrates

Simple and complex carbohydrates are two sub-categories of carbohydrates.

Simple carbohydrates include monosaccharides and disaccharides. Complex carbohydrates are long chains of monosaccharides. Complex carbohydrates include starch and fibers.

Simple carbohydrate is also called fast-releasing carbohydrate, and complex carbohydrate is called slow-releasing carbohydrate.

Simple carbohydrates include monosaccharides and disaccharides.

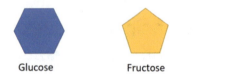

Glucose, fructose, and galactose are monosaccharides.

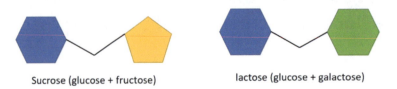

Sucrose and Lactose are Disaccharides.

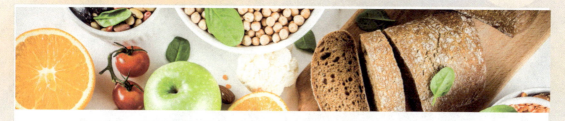

Simple carbohydrates

Simple carbohydrates are also known as "sugars" and are grouped as either monosaccharides or disaccharides. Monosaccharides include glucose, fructose, and galactose, and disaccharides include lactose, maltose, and sucrose.

Simple carbohydrates stimulate the sweet taste sensation, the most sensitive of all taste sensations. Even low concentrations of sugars in foods will stimulate the sweet taste sensation. Sweetness varies between the different carbohydrate types—some are much sweeter than others. Fructose is the top naturally occurring sugar in sweetness value.

The illustration of simple carbohydrates:
monosaccharides and disaccharides

Glucose Fructose Galactose

Monosaccharides:
glucose, fructose, and galactose

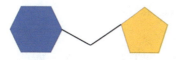

Sucrose (glucose + fructose)

Disaccharides:
sucrose and lactose

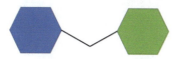

lactose (glucose + galactose)

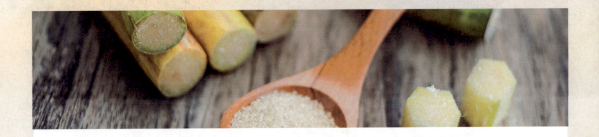

Monosaccharides

In addition to glucose, there are two other monosaccharides, galactose and fructose, most often in the human diet.

For plants and animals, glucose is the preferred fuel source. The human brain depends on glucose, except during extreme starvation conditions.

Galactose is a monosaccharide sugar. Galactose is found in avocados, sugar beets, and dairy products. The body also synthesizes it. Galactose is utilized for energy production in cells after converting to glucose. A galactose molecule unit linked with a glucose unit forms lactose, the natural sugar in milk.

Fructose is a monosaccharide that is primarily found in fruits. Fructose is among the most common monosaccharides in nature. It is also found in some drinks, cereals, and other products sweetened with fructose-containing corn syrup.

Simple carbohydrates

Monosaccharides are simple carbohydrates.

Monosaccharides: "Mono" means "one"; "saccharide" means "sugar."

Monosaccharides are carbohydrates in their most basic form.

Monosaccharides in the human diet include glucose, fructose, and galactose.

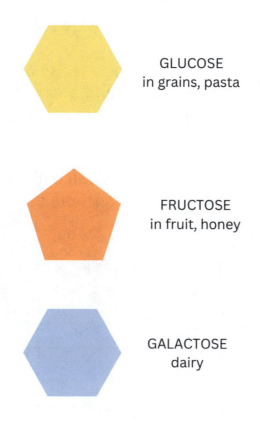

GLUCOSE
in grains, pasta

FRUCTOSE
in fruit, honey

GALACTOSE
dairy

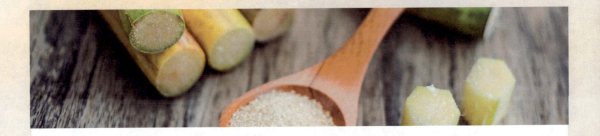

Disaccharides

Our daily diet has three main types of disaccharides: sucrose, lactose, and maltose.

Sucrose is a disaccharide, the sugar sold in the grocery store as table sugar, icing sugar, or granular sugar. Each sucrose molecule comprises one unit of glucose and one unit of fructose. Sucrose is found in many fruits and vegetables and in high concentrations in sugarcane and sugar beets, used to extract sucrose sold as table sugar in grocery stores.

Lactose, commonly known as milk sugar, comprises one glucose unit and one galactose unit in each lactose molecule. Lactose is prevalent in dairy products such as cheese, yogurt, and milk.

Maltose is a disaccharide. Two molecules of glucose fuse to form each maltose molecule. Maltose is produced in the seeds and roots of plants as they break down the stored energy and nutrients to sprout. Thus, maltose is contained naturally in high amounts in foods like cereals, sweet potatoes, and certain fruits.

Disaccharides

When two monosaccharides bind chemically, they form a disaccharide.

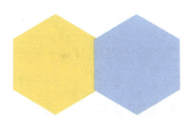

Lactose (from dairy) is a disaccharide synthesized by one galactose + one glucose subunit.

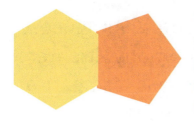

Sucrose (from sugar beet and cane sugar) is a disaccharide composed of glucose and fructose subunits. It is produced naturally in plants and is the main constituent of white sugar.

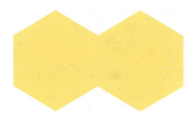

Maltose (from molasses, beer). Maltose is a disaccharide formed from two units of glucose joined together.

Glucose

Glucose is the most abundant simple sugar found in nature. Glucose is found in honey, other sweeteners, fruits, and other plant foods. Plants make their glucose for energy.

Glucose is humans' primary energy source as well. Most of our carbohydrates are digested into glucose for the body to use. The amount of glucose in our blood is referred to as blood glucose or blood sugar, which is vital to the proper functioning of our bodies. As glucose travels in the blood around the body, it enters cells and is used as fuel. Glucose is also part of all double sugars, starches, and fibres.

Glucose

Glucose

Glucose, the blood sugar, and the mechanism of glucose regulation in our bodies.

Glucose is the main carbohydrate used for energy, and glucose circulates in the bloodstream. It is often called blood glucose. It is carried to all body cells. Each cell has its powerhouse, which uses blood glucose to fuel the cell.

When carbohydrates are absorbed, blood glucose levels rise. The hormone secreted by the pancreas, Insulin, helps glucose enter cells, where it is used for energy.

However, the body does not turn all blood glucose into energy at once. As blood glucose levels rise above average, Insulin signals the liver, muscles, and some other cells to store the extra; some get stored in the muscles and liver as glycogen, a carbohydrate storage form composed of many connected glucose molecules. Some glucose may be converted to body fat if more carbohydrate is consumed than the body use or burns. That's why it is suggested to keep your carbs intake under control to keep a check on body fat.

When blood glucose levels drop below normal, another hormone called glucagon triggers the conversion of glycogen to glucose. This is how blood glucose levels stay within a normal range between meals. Once glucose is in your bloodstream, it fuels body cells.

The human body also obtains energy from fat and protein. However, carbohydrate is the primary energy source. Fat becomes an energy source when the body does not have enough carbohydrates for energy. In addition, if your calorie intake is less than what your body needs and if the limited glycogen stores are used up, body proteins are broken down for energy. Getting enough carbs from food choices can spare or save protein for what only protein can do: build and repair body cells and tissues.

Glucose

Glucose & Serotonin

Glucose is the preferred energy source for muscles during strenuous exercise. When the body's glucose supply is depleted, it turns to fat for energy. The body also requires glucose to fuel multiple unconscious biological processes.

Glucose is essential fuel for the brain, aiding in concentration. In addition, carbohydrates are critical for generating the brain's serotonin supply. Serotonin is a mood-regulating hormone made by our bodies from tryptophan; tryptophan is an amino acid obtained through protein in the diet.

Carbohydrates help convert tryptophan into serotonin; eating carbs may help enhance mood. This suggests that carbs and sweet foods are often treated as comfort foods. In addition, serotonin is converted to melatonin, a hormone that helps regulate circadian rhythm.

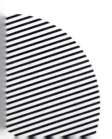

Serotonin, the happy hormone

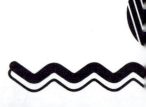

Melatonin, the hormone that helps regulate circadian rhythm.

Fructose, the fruit sugar, is a monosaccharide.

Fructose, the sweetest natural sugar, is found in fruits and honey. Fructose is a monosaccharide. Fructose is also known as fruit sugar, as fructose primarily occurs naturally in many fruits. Fructose is also contained naturally in other plant-based foods such as honey, sugar cane, sugar beets, and vegetables.

Fructose, or fruit sugar, is a simple sugar found in many plants, where it is often bonded to glucose to form the disaccharide sucrose. Fructose, glucose, and galactose are the three dietary monosaccharides absorbed by the gut directly into the liver after digestion through the portal vein. The liver then converts fructose and galactose into glucose, so dissolved glucose, also known as blood sugar, is the only monosaccharide in circulating blood.

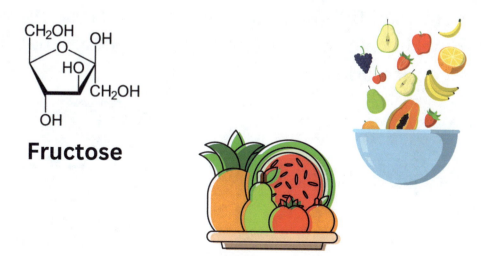

Fructose

Sucrose | the sugar, also called icing sugar, table sugar, granulated sugar | sucrose is a disaccharide.

Sucrose, a disaccharide, is a sugar composed of one glucose and one fructose sub-unit in each sucrose molecule. Sucrose is commonly called white sugar, table sugar, or simply sugar. Sucrose is the chemical name of the double sugar containing glucose and fructose. Sucrose is merely two common single sugars-glucose and fructose-linked together.

Sucrose occurs naturally in small amounts in many fruits and vegetables. It is produced naturally in plants and is mainly found in sugar cane, therefore called cane sugar. Sucrose is extracted and refined from either sugar cane or sugar beet. Food sugar is often sucrose, added to soft drinks, cookies, cakes, and other pastries. White sugar is sucrose and is more than 99% pure sucrose, and sucrose provides four kilocalories per gram but no other nutrients except calories.

sucrose

Lactose, a disaccharide, is the natural sugar in milk.

Although milk is not a food you think of as sweet, milk contains sugar lactose. Lactose is a natural sugar contained in milk and milk products, like cheese and yogurt, and lactose is only slightly sweet.

Lactose is a disaccharide, and one lactose molecule shall consist of two simple sugar units, a glucose molecule unit, and a galactose molecule unit. Lactose makes up around 2–8% of milk. Lactose is one of the lowest-ranking sugars in terms of sweetness. Lactose is also the only sugar found naturally in animal products.

Lactose (from dairy) is a disaccharide synthesized by one galactose + one glucose subunit.

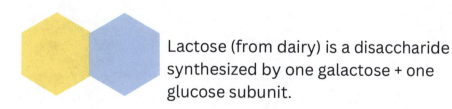

lactose

Starch and fiber, the polysaccharides

Starches and fibers are also called complex carbohydrates because they are made of long chains of glucose, as plants store glucose in the form of starch. Starch is a natural component of most plants, fruits, grains, and vegetables. Starch is also called polysaccharides, and each starch molecule is composed of numerous glucose units joined together. Most green plants produce this polysaccharide for energy storage.

In human bodies, glycogen is the energy reserve; glycogen is a highly branched version of starch. Starch is a polysaccharide comprising glucose monomers joined together to form long-molecular chains.

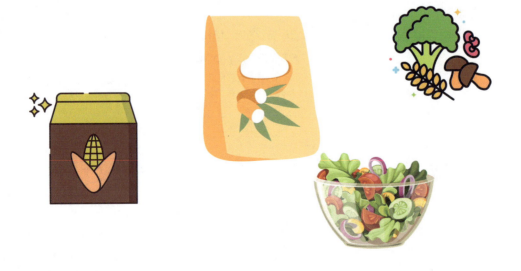

Starch and Fibers

Starch and fibres are carbohydrates and polysaccharides; they have long chains composed of glucose molecule units.

Starch and fibre often need clarification since both are contained in the same foods and with macromolecular structures. In starch, chains of glucose monomers (monomer means one single molecule) are joined by alpha bonds, which can be broken down in the small intestine. In fibre, glucose monomers are joined by beta bonds, which can not be broken down; instead, the chains remain intact throughout their passage through the small intestine.

Starch
starch like amylopectin, found in potato, rice, bread and pasta, wheat and barley) are made with alpha-glucose monomers. The bond angles are formed when alpha-glucose monomers join a branched or spiral structure. These bonds can be broken down by enzymes in the digestive system.

Fiber
Polysaccharides like cellulose in plants are made with beta-glucose monomers. The bond angles are formed when glucose units join and build into stable, strongly interlinked parallel chains. Enzymes in the small intestine can not break down these beta-bonds in fibres.

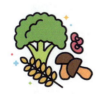 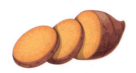

Starch: In starch, alpha glucose is the monomer unit. As a result of the bond angles in the alpha-acetal linkage, starch (amylose) forms a spiral and branched structure.

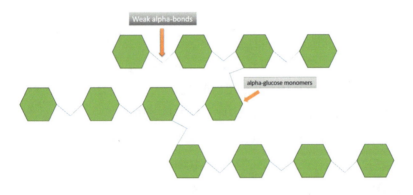

Starch

Fiber such as Cellulose:
As a result of the bond angles in the beta-acetal linkage, cellulose is primarily a linear chain.

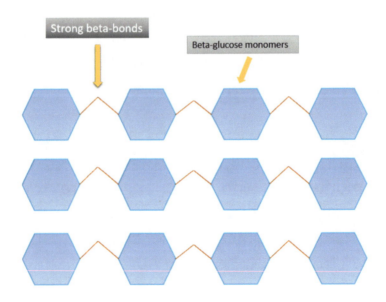

Fibre

Starchy foods are the body's primary source of energy.

Starchy foods are essential to a balanced diet, providing energy, fibre, and a sense of fullness. The body breaks down starch molecules into glucose, the body's primary fuel source.

Grains are the seeds of cultivated grasses. Examples of grains are wheat, corn, rice, rye, barley, and oats. Wheat flour bakes bread and many other baked goods and makes cereals, crackers, and pasta.

Naturally, starch accumulates in the roots and tubers of various vegetables, providing energy for the plant to grow. Examples of roots and tubers include potatoes and sweet potatoes, which provide much starch for people. Dried beans and peas, such as beans and split peas, are also rich starch sources.

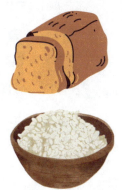
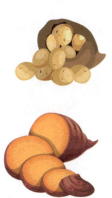

Starch

Starches, complex carbohydrates

Starches and fibres are two groups of polysaccharides. Polysaccharides are long chains of monosaccharides. Polysaccharides are also called complex carbohydrates.

Starch molecules are abundant in grains, legumes, and root vegetables, such as potatoes. Isolated and modified starches are used widely in the food industry and during cooking as food thickeners.

Resistant starches are the term defining the starches that remain intact throughout digestion. Bacteria in the gut can break some of these down. Resistant starches have potential gastrointestinal benefits as they provide bulk volume and satiety to food, promote bowel movements, and add no calories.

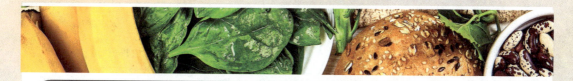

Dietary Fibers

Humans do not produce the enzymes that break down dietary fiber; however, large intestine (colon) bacteria can break down some fibers. Dietary fibers are beneficial to our health. Studies show that diets high in fiber may reduce some obesity and obesity-related health risks.

Water-soluble dietary fiber and water-insoluble dietary fiber

Dietary fiber is categorized as water-soluble or insoluble, depending on whether it dissolves in water. Soluble fibers are found in beans, peas, oats, barley, and rye. Soluble fibers include inulin, pectin, and guar gum.

Insoluble fibers include cellulose and lignin, which are not soluble in water. The dietary sources of insoluble fibers include whole grains, flax, cauliflower, and avocados. Cellulose is the most abundant fiber in plants, making up the cell walls and providing cell structure.

Soluble fibers are more easily accessible to bacterial enzymes in the large intestine, so they can be broken down more than insoluble fibers. For example, some cellulose and other insoluble fibers breakdown occurs in the large intestine.

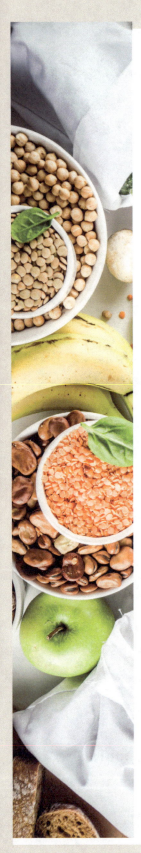

Fiber, the carbohydrate

Fibre is a carbohydrate that human digestive enzymes cannot completely break down. Unlike other types of carbohydrates, most fibers can not be broken down into glucose and used by the body as an energy source. Instead, fiber passes through the body undigested. However, fiber helps regulate the body's use of sugars, helping to keep hunger and blood sugar in check. In addition, fiber helps improve the health of the digestive tract.

Like starch, most dietary fibers are long chains of glucose. But what is different is that our digestive systems lack the enzymes to break apart the bond that connects the glucose in fiber, as the bond between the glucose in the fiber chains differs from the bond in starch. The net result is that fiber can not be broken down in our digestive tract, so it passes through the stomach and intestines unchanged and then is excreted.

Fiber is abundant in plants. Most natural foods contain a variety of fibers. Good sources of fiber include legumes, fruits, vegetables, nuts, and seeds, and foods made from grains such as flour, rice, and brown rice.

Dietary fiber has two main components: soluble fiber and insoluble fiber, which are components of plant-based foods such as legumes, whole grains, cereals, nuts, or seeds.

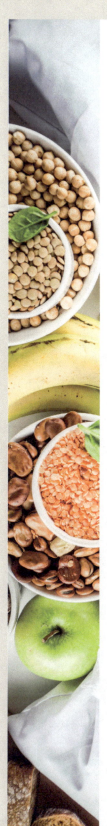

Soluble fiber

Soluble fiber swells in water and becomes sticky and gummy. Because of this, soluble fibers slow down the digestive process and, therefore, suppress hunger. This makes us feel full longer after eating. This hunger-suppressing effect of soluble fibers facilitates weight loss through a better eating timetable pattern and refraining from heavy snacks.

Soluble fibers are also beneficial because they bond cholesterol compounds in the intestines and carry them out of the body. Plant foods rich in soluble fiber include beans, oats, apples, citrus fruits, and some vegetables such as broccoli, Brussels sprouts, and sweet potatoes.

Soluble fibers provide a food source for some intestinal bacteria, which is good because these bacteria help keep the intestine healthy. When bacteria digest fiber, they produce small amounts of fatty acids that are absorbed into the body.

Insoluble fiber

Insoluble fiber is a dietary fiber that can not be dissolved in water.

Insoluble fiber is helpful for people with constipation because this type of fiber softens stool and helps food pass through the digestive tract more quickly. Plant foods rich in insoluble fiber include wheat bran, beans, peas, lentils, whole grains, whole wheat, and many vegetables and fruits.

Apples' dietary fiber illustration

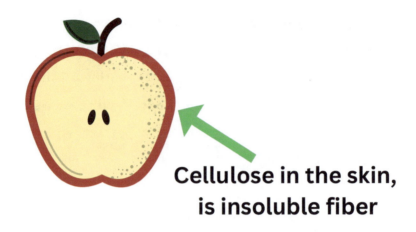

Cellulose in the skin, is insoluble fiber

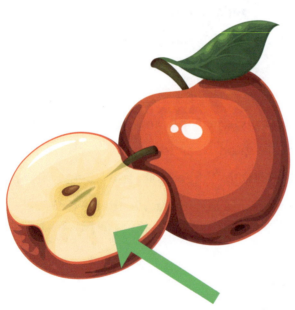

Pectin.
water-soluble colloidal fibers

The following table summarizes a few types of natural fibers that you may see in the current market.

The naturally occurring plant fibers

fiber	source	function
Lignins	Insoluble fiber is found in wheat and corn bran, nuts, flaxseeds, vegetables, and unripe bananas.	Triggers mucus secretion in the colon and adds bulk to stools.
Beta-glucans	The soluble, highly fermentable fiber found in oats and barley	Beta-glucans are metabolized and fermented in the small intestine. It acts as a prebiotic. Can add bulk to stool. It may help to normalize blood glucose and cholesterol levels.
Guar gum	Guar gum is water-soluble fermentable fiber isolated from guar beans. Guar gum has thickening and stabilizing properties useful in food industry applications.	It has a viscous gel texture and is often added to foods as a thickener. It is metabolized and fermented in the small intestine. It may help to normalize blood sugar and cholesterol levels.

The following table summarizes a few types of natural fibers that you may see in the current market.

The naturally occurring plant fibers

Fiber	Source	Function
Inulin	Soluble, fermentable fibers are found in onions, chicory roots, and asparagus.	Inulin acts as a prebiotic. Inulin is not digested or absorbed in the stomach. Inulin stays in the bowel and functions as food feeding certain beneficial bacteria to grow. Inulin is a starchy substance existing in a variety of fruits and vegetables.
Pectins	The soluble, highly fermentable fiber is found in apples, berries, and other fruits.	Pectins' gelling properties may slow digestion and help normalize blood sugar and cholesterol levels.
Resistant starch	Resistant starch is a fermentable fiber found in legumes, bananas, cooked and cooled pasta, and potatoes that act as a prebiotic.	Humans can not digest resistant starch in the small intestine. Instead, resistant starch ferments in the large intestine and feeds "good" gut bacteria.
Cellulose and hemicellulose	Insoluble fiber is found in cereal grains and the cell walls of many fruits and vegetables.	It absorbs water and adds bulk to stool.

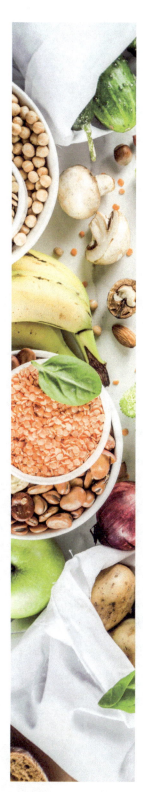

Carbohydrates and Energy

Carbohydrates are critical to support life's most basic function—energy production. Without energy, none of the life processes can be performed. As the primary energy source, carbohydrates must be consumed in moderation to provide energy to perform all functions and activities.

Carbohydrates for Energy Production

The primary role of carbohydrates is to supply energy to all cells in the body. Many cells prefer glucose as an energy source versus other compounds like fatty acids. Some cells, such as red blood cells, can only produce cellular energy from glucose.

When glucose is insufficient to meet the body's needs, glucose is synthesized from amino acids; amino acids are the building blocks for protein. The presence of adequate glucose spares the breakdown of proteins, which can be used to build body muscle, soft tissues, and other functional uses.

Carbohydrates aid in lipid Metabolism.

Glucose has a fat-sparing effect, as when blood glucose levels rise, the use of lipids as an energy source is inhibited. An increase in blood glucose stimulates the release of the hormone insulin, which tells cells to use glucose instead of lipids to make energy.

Glycogen, Carbohydrates for Energy Storage

> **Glycogen, the energy storage in the body**

The excess glucose is stored as glycogen if the body has enough energy to support its functions. Most of the glycogen is stored in the muscles and the liver. A glycogen molecule may contain fifty thousand single glucose units and is highly branched, allowing for the rapid dissemination of glucose when needed to make cellular energy.

Muscles can store glycogen as an energy source. Prolonged muscle use, such as protracted exercise for more than a few hours, can deplete the glycogen energy reserve. After a lengthy workout, muscle glycogen is consumed, and muscles must rely more on proteins and lipids as energy sources.

The liver can store glucose energy as glycogen. The liver uses its stored glycogen to support other bodily tissues when blood glucose levels are low. Approximately a quarter of total body glycogen content is in the liver, equivalent to about a four-hour supply of glucose, but this is highly dependent on activity level.

The liver uses this glycogen reserve to keep blood glucose levels within a narrow range between meal times. When the liver's glycogen supply is exhausted, glucose is made from amino acids obtained from destroying proteins to maintain body functions.

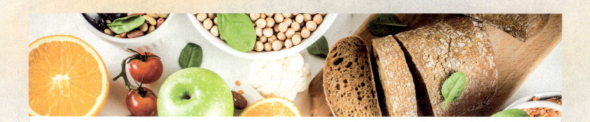

More about carbohydrates

Carbohydrates from plant-based foods

Carbohydrates are the ideal nutrient to meet your body's nutritional needs. Carbohydrates nourish the brain and nervous system, provide energy to all your cells within proper caloric limits, and help keep the body fit.

Specifically, digestible carbohydrates provide bulk in foods, vitamins, and minerals, while indigestible carbohydrates provide good fiber and other health benefits.

Plants harness the sun's energy to synthesize glucose from carbon dioxide in the air and water. Plants convert the energy in sunlight to chemical energy in glucose. This is called photosynthesis. Glucose is a fast-releasing carbohydrate that can be directly used for energy in plants and humans. Plants use glucose to make other larger, more slow-releasing carbohydrates, starches, and fibers. When we eat plant foods, we harvest the energy of glucose, starches, fibers, and other phytonutrients from plant-based foods to support our life processes.

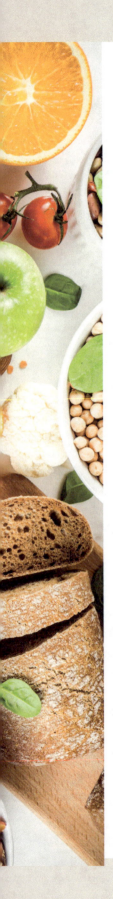

Digestion and Absorption of Carbohydrates

From the Mouth to the Stomach

The digestion of carbohydrates starts from eating the foods as the chemical and mechanical digestion of carbohydrates begins in the mouth.

The Chewing Process crumbles the carbohydrate foods into smaller pieces. The saliva secreted from the salivary glands coats the food to facilitate absorption.

About five percent of starches in foods are broken down in the mouth with the aid of amylase enzyme in saliva. No further chemical breakdown of starches occurs once carbohydrates reach the stomach because the amylase enzyme in saliva does not function in the acidic conditions of the stomach. However, the mechanical breakdown of starches continues as the powerful peristaltic contractions of the stomach mix the food into a more uniform mixture called chyme.

From the Stomach to the Small Intestine

From the stomach, the chyme is gradually expelled into the upper part of the small intestine. Upon the chyme's entry into the small intestine, the pancreatic juice joins in to help break down the carbohydrates into single sugar, which are then transported into intestinal cells.

Digestion and Absorption of Carbohydrates

Absorption of carbohydrate: Going to the Blood Stream

The small intestine cells have membranes containing many transport proteins to get the monosaccharides and other nutrients into the blood, which can be distributed to the rest of the body. The carbohydrates we eat are digested into simple sugars like glucose, fructose, and galactose.

The liver is the first organ to receive glucose, fructose, and galactose. The liver breaks fructose into smaller carbon-containing units and converts galactose to glucose. The final product from the digestion of carbohydrates is glucose, which is either used for energy or stored as triglyceride in fat or glycogen in muscle and liver. The liver either stores glucose as glycogen or exports glucose to the blood.

Glycogen in the liver and muscles

Humans and animals store glucose energy from starches in the form of the very large molecule glycogen. It has many branches that allow it to break down quickly when energy is needed by cells in the body. It is predominantly found in the liver and muscle tissue in animals.

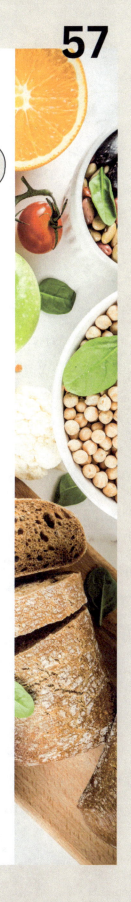

Digestion and Absorption of Carbohydrates

Maintaining Blood Glucose Levels

The blood glucose level is tightly controlled by the synergy of various hormones, organs, and tissues in our bodies, as having either too much or too little glucose in the blood can have severe health consequences.

One of the glucose regulators in our bodies is located in the cells of the pancreas. After eating carbohydrates, glucose level rises in the blood. The increase in blood glucose level is sensed by pancreas insulin-secreting cells, which then release insulin into the blood. Insulin is a hormone made by the pancreas that helps glucose in blood enter cells in muscle, liver, and fat, where it is used or stored. In muscle tissue and the liver, insulin sends the biological message to store glucose as glycogen.

Insulin in the blood signifies to the body cells that glucose is available for fuel. Insulin signals the body's cells to remove glucose from the blood. Blood glucose levels decrease as glucose is transported into the cells around the body. Insulin has an opposing hormone called glucagon. The pancreas also produces glucagon. Glucagon-secreting cells in the pancreas sense the drop in glucose and, in response, release glucagon into the blood. Glucagon stimulates increases in blood sugar levels, thus opposing the action of insulin. Glucagon signals the liver to break down glycogen and release the stored glucose into the blood so that glucose levels stay within the target range and all cells get the needed fuel to function normally.

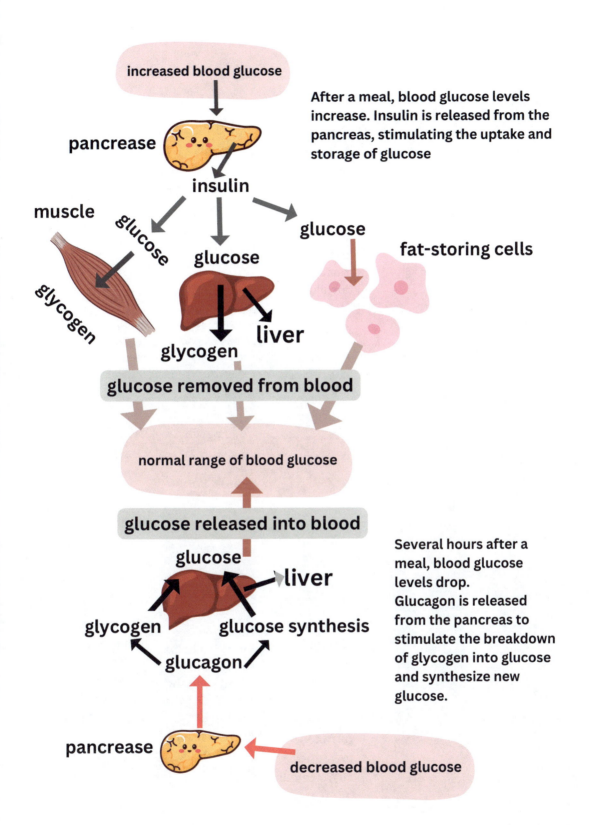

Pancreatic cells

The pancreatic islets also referred to as the islets of Langerhans, are clusters of cells that secrete the hormones responsible for balancing metabolism. These hormones balance blood sugar levels as the body oscillates between the fed and fasted states.

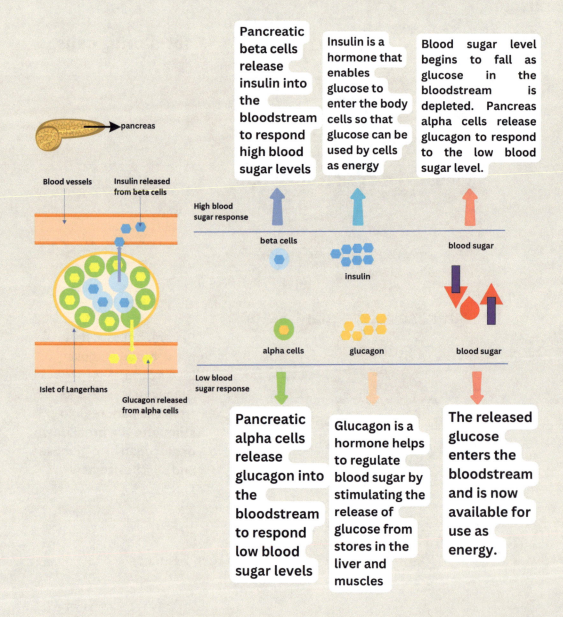

Digesting carbohydrates

The less starchy complex carbohydrates are broken down into simple carbohydrates in the small intestine.
All non-glucose monosaccharides are converted into glucose in the liver and released into the bloodstream. It is used immediately or converted into glycogen, a polysaccharide of glucose stored in the liver and muscles for later use.

Fibre refers to any complex carbohydrates that can not be broken down by the digestive enzymes in the small intestine. This fibrous matter moves into the large intestine, where it helps produce beneficial short-chain fatty acids and nourishes the lining of the gut.

Generally, carbohydrates in their natural, fiber-rich form are more nutritious than those stripped of their fiber content. Fruits and vegetables are excellent sources of carbohydrates.

Overview of Carbohydrate Digestion

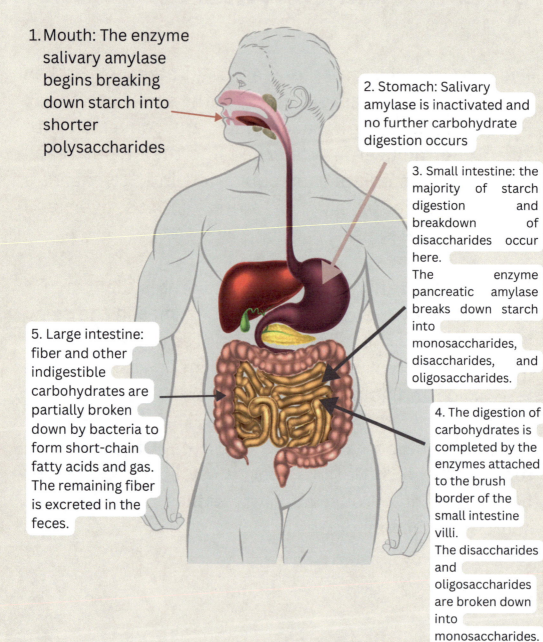

1. Mouth: The enzyme salivary amylase begins breaking down starch into shorter polysaccharides

2. Stomach: Salivary amylase is inactivated and no further carbohydrate digestion occurs

3. Small intestine: the majority of starch digestion and breakdown of disaccharides occur here.
The enzyme pancreatic amylase breaks down starch into monosaccharides, disaccharides, and oligosaccharides.

4. The digestion of carbohydrates is completed by the enzymes attached to the brush border of the small intestine villi.
The disaccharides and oligosaccharides are broken down into monosaccharides.

5. Large intestine: fiber and other indigestible carbohydrates are partially broken down by bacteria to form short-chain fatty acids and gas. The remaining fiber is excreted in the feces.

Fiber digestion in the large intestine

Almost all carbohydrates, except dietary fiber and resistant starches, are efficiently digested and absorbed into the body. Some of the remaining indigestible carbohydrates are broken down by enzymes released by bacteria in the large intestine. The products of bacterial digestion of these slow-releasing carbohydrates are short-chain fatty acids and some gases. The yield of energy from the dietary fiber is about two calories per gram but is highly dependent upon the fiber type, with soluble fibers and resistant starches yielding more energy than insoluble fibers. Since dietary fiber is digested much less in the gastrointestinal tract than other carbohydrate types (simple sugars, many starches), the rise in blood glucose after eating them is less and slower. These physiological attributes of high-fiber foods like whole grains are linked to a reduction in weight gain and reduced risk of chronic diseases, such as Type 2 diabetes and cardiovascular diseases.

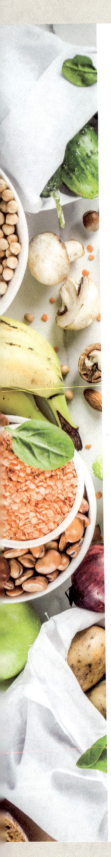

It's the Whole Nutrient Package

In choosing dietary sources of carbohydrates, the best choices are those that are nutrient-dense, meaning they contain more essential nutrients per kilocalorie of energy. Nutrient-dense carbohydrates are minimally processed, including whole-grain bread and cereals, low-fat dairy products, fruits, vegetables, and beans.

In contrast, empty-calorie carbohydrate foods are highly processed and often contain added sugars and saturated fats. Empty-calorie carbohydrates include soft drinks, cakes, cookies, and candy. They are sometimes called 'bad carbohydrates,' as they have no other significant nutrients except added sugar.

Reference: Part D. Section 5: Carbohydrates. In Report of the DGAC on the Dietary Guidelines for Americans, US Department of Agriculture. 2010.

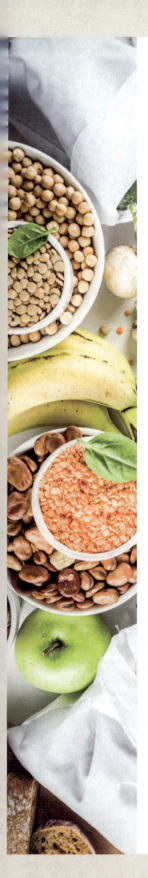

The calories of carbohydrates, sugar, and starch.

Whether from sugars or starch, a single gram of carbohydrate fuels your body with the same amount of energy, four kilocalories per gram of sugar or starches. By comparison, protein supplies four kilocalories per gram, and fat provides nine kilocalories per gram.

Fiber fermentation in the gut is estimated to provide two kilocalories per gram of dietary fiber. However, since not all fiber is fermentable, calculating fiber's energy value poses problems and can lead to calorie miscalculations.

The bottom line of carbohydrates is : For your health, make nutrient-rich carbohydrate foods your body's primary energy source.

Reference:

Institute of Medicine 2005. Dietary Reference Intakes for Energy, Carbohydrates, Fiber, Fat, Fatty Acids, Cholesterol, Protein, and Amino Acids. Washington, DC: The National Academies Press. https://doi.org/10.17226/10490.

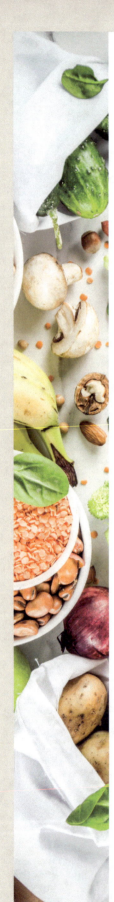

Glycemic Index- A helpful tool for Diabetics

The Glycemic Index(GI) is a number or value that tells about the rise in blood glucose level after eating a specific food. Different foods have different Glycemic Index Values. Foods are classified into three categories based on their GI values and ranked on a scale of 0-100.

Here are the three GI ratings:
- Low: 55 or less
- Medium: 56–69
- High: 70 or above

Foods having low GI values have little effect on blood sugar levels, while High GI foods have a high effect on blood glucose levels.

Thus, Diabetics shall choose low-GI foods to better control their blood glucose levels.

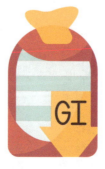

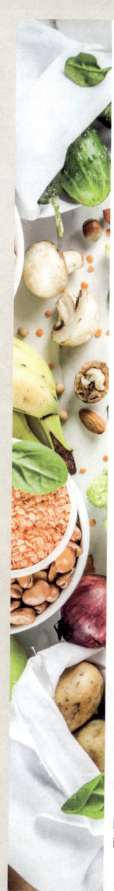

Glycemic Load (GL)- A tool to control Blood Glucose Levels

Glycemic Load(GL) measures how much blood glucose levels will rise after eating a certain amount of food.

GL tells us about the amount of Carbohydrates in our food and how much one gram of that food will raise our blood glucose levels. The Glycemic Load helps us know about the Carbs portion of our meals.

Thus, Glycemic Index and Glycemic Load are beneficial tools for controlling blood glucose levels. The difference is that Glycemic Load is specific to the amount of food, while Glycemic load does not consider the amount of food.

Calculating glycaemic load (GL)

The GL calculation is GI x the amount of carbohydrates (in grams) in a serving of food) ÷ 100.

For example:
 An apple (GI = 40, carbohydrate = 15g).
GL of an apple = 40 x 15/100 = 6g.

References:
https://www.mayoclinic.org/diseases-conditions/diabetes/expert-answers/diabetes/faq-20058466

https://www.healthline.com/nutrition/glycemic-index#what-it-is

https://www.health.harvard.edu/diseases-and-conditions/the-lowdown-on-glycemic-index-and-glycemic-load

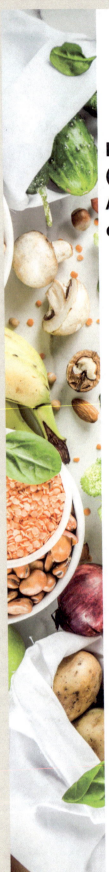

Low Glycemic Index (55 or less) food A short list of example foods

- apple
- berries
- cantaloupe
- grapefruit
- honeydew melon
- orange
- peach
- pear
- pomegranate
- chickpeas
- kidney beans
- lentils
- mung beans
- soybeans

Medium Glycemic Index (56 to 69) food A short list of example foods

- grapes
- lychee
- pineapple
- raisins
- white rice
- brown rice
- cornmeal
- rice noodles

High Glycemic Index (70 or more) food A short list of example foods:

- bread (white and whole wheat)
- Jasmine rice
- millet
- sticky rice
- Hot potato (red and white)

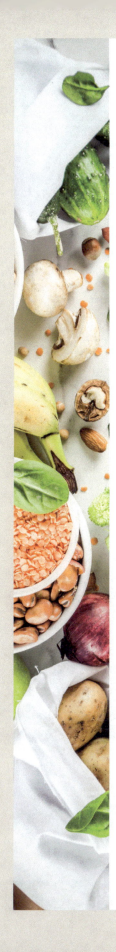

Empty calories

Saturated fats and added sugars enhance the flavors and tastes of foods when cooking the foods and make the foods more appealing. Nowadays, many foods and beverages contain empty calories, which means calories from saturated fats or added sugars that add few or no nutrients. Saturated fats and added sugars contribute about 35% of daily calories without contributing to the overall nutrient adequacy of the diet.

Saturated fats are found naturally in foods or added when foods are prepared at home or processed by food companies. Saturated fats usually are solid at room temperature. Coconut oil and palm oil are high in saturated fats.

Added sugars are sugars like white sugar that are added to a food for sweetening and flavor (such as soda and cookies) or added to foods or beverages at the table. Increased consumption of added sugars increases the risk of becoming obese and is a factor in rising obesity rates among adults and children. However, sugars found naturally in fruits and dairy products are not added sugars. You don't need to eliminate saturated fats or added sugars from your diet, but you need to moderate your intake of them.

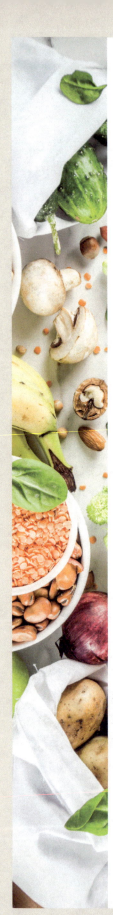

Sugar Substitutes to lessen empty calories in the diet

Sugar substitutes are artificial sweeteners or natural sweeteners extracted from plants. Sugar substitutes usually give a sweet taste to foods and beverages while providing little or no calories.

In this book, we have given you a general description of sugar substitutes, including artificial sweeteners and natural sugar substitutes. In this book, we have explained three sweeteners: saccharin, sucralose, and stevia.

Sugar Substitutes

Sugar substitutes, also known as artificial sweeteners or sugar alternatives, are synthetic or natural compounds that are used to sweeten foods and beverages and provide little or no calories. These sweeteners have become increasingly popular in recent years as people seek to reduce their sugar intake for various reasons, including managing weight, controlling blood sugar levels, and maintaining overall health. Sugar substitutes provide a sweet taste without the negative effects of excessive sugar consumption, such as tooth decay and spikes in blood sugar.

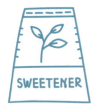

Sugar Substitutes

Artificial sweeteners are specifically designed to mimic the taste of sugar, often many times sweeter than sugar itself, so only a tiny amount is needed to achieve the desired level of sweetness. They are widely used in many products, including diet sodas, sugar-free candies, and low-calorie desserts. Common artificial sweeteners include Saccharin(brand names: Sweet 'N Low and Sugar Twin), Aspartame(brand names: Equal and NutraSweet Natural), Sucralose(brand names: Splenda), Neotame(brand name: Newtame), and Acesulfame potassium(brand names: Sunett and Sweet One), each with its unique taste profile and uses.

Natural sugar substitutes, on the other hand, are derived from plant sources and are considered a more natural alternative to artificial sweeteners. Examples of Natural sugar substitutes include Steviol glycosides (found in stevia plants), Sugar alcohols (Erythritol, Lactitol, Mannitol, Maltitol, Sorbitol, and Xylitol), Allulose(found in fruits), Honey, Molasses, and monk fruit extract. These options often have fewer or no calories and may have additional health benefits, such as potential antioxidant properties or a lower impact on blood sugar levels.

The use of sugar substitutes and artificial sweeteners has generated both excitement and debate within the food industry and among health-conscious consumers. While they can be a valuable tool for reducing sugar consumption and managing certain health conditions, some people have concerns about potential long-term health effects or their impact on taste preferences. It's essential to use sugar substitutes in moderation and consult with a healthcare professional if you have specific dietary or health concerns related to their use.

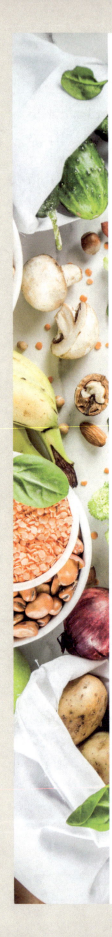

Sugar Substitutes

We introduce three popular sweeteners in this book:
- **Saccharin;**
- **Sucralose;**
- **Stevia.**

Saccharin:

Saccharin, also called saccharine or benzosulfimide, Saccharin has brand names Sweet'N Low and Sugar Twin.
Its Melting Point is in the range of 228.8 to 229.7 °C (443.8 to 445.5 °F; 501.9 to 502.8 K)

Saccharin is a benzoic sulfimide that is about 500 times sweeter than sucrose but has a bitter or metallic aftertaste, especially at high concentrations. It is used to sweeten products, such as drinks, candies, baked goods, tobacco products, and excipients, and mask the bitter taste of some medicines. It appears as white crystals and is odorless.
It is considered stable and safe within the temperature range typically encountered in food and beverage preparation and storage, which is generally from room temperature to the boiling point of water (0°C to 100°C or 32°F to 212°F).

Saccharin's decomposition temperature, the temperature at which it starts to break down, is higher than the typical temperatures used in cooking and baking. The decomposition temperature of saccharin is approximately 228°C (442°F).

Saccharin has no food energy and no nutritional value. It is safe to consume for individuals with diabetes or prediabetes. Saccharin was associated with bladder cancer and was banned by the FDA and in many other countries. However, recent research doesn't support this claim. The current status of saccharin is that it is allowed in most countries, and countries such as Canada have lifted their previous ban on it as a food additive.

Reference:
https://en.wikipedia.org/wiki/Saccharin

Saccharin

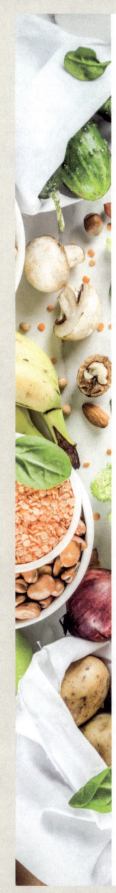

Sugar Substitutes

73

Sucralose:

Sucralose is sold under the brand name **Splenda®**.
Its chemical name is ortho-benzoic sulfimide.
Its melting point is 125 °C (257 °F; 398 K).

Sucralose is about 320 to 1,000 times sweeter than sucrose. The body does not break down the majority of ingested sucralose, so it is noncaloric. While sucralose is largely considered shelf-stable and safe for use at elevated temperatures (such as in baked goods), there is some evidence that it begins to break down at temperatures above 119 °C (246 °F).

Sucralose was first approved to be used in Canada in 1991 and in the US in 1998. In 2006, the FDA amended food regulations to include sucralose as a "non-nutritive sweetener" in food.

Reference:
https://en.wikipedia.org/wiki/Sucralose

Sucralose

Sugar Substitutes

Stevia

Stevia is a sweet sugar substitute extracted from the leaves of the plant species Stevia rebaudiana native to Paraguay and Brazil. The active compounds are steviol glycosides, which have about 50 to 300 times the sweetness of sugar and are heat-stable, pH-stable, and not fermentable. The human body does not metabolize the glycosides in stevia, so it contains zero calories as a non-nutritive sweetener. Stevia lends itself well to cooking and baking, unlike some artificial and chemical sweeteners that break down at higher temperatures. Stevia is stable at temperatures of up to 392° Fahrenheit (200° Celsius) making it an ideal sugar substitute (with some adjustments) for many recipes.

In the United States, certain high-purity stevia glycoside extracts have been generally recognized as safe (GRAS) and may be lawfully marketed and added to food products but Stevia leaf and crude extracts do not have GRAS or Food and Drug Administration (FDA) approval for use in food. A popular brand of stevia powder is PureVia.

References:
1. https://www.stevia.org/stevia-recipes/cooking-with-stevia#:~:text=Stevia%20is%20stable%20at%20temperatures%20of%20up%20to,sugar%20substitute%20%28with%20some%20adjustments%29%20for%20many%20recipes.

2. https://en.wikipedia.org/wiki/Stevia

stevioside, one type of steviol glycoside

Fats

Fat is one of the six groups of nutrients required by human bodies to function normally. Fats and cholesterol are members of a group of compounds called lipids. Fats are the most abundant lipids in nature and are found in plants and animals. A lipid is customarily called a fat if it is a solid at room temperature and an oil if it is a liquid at room temperature.

Fats in foods are usually from animal sources, such as butter and beef fat, whereas oils are generally of plant origin. We commonly speak of animal fats and vegetable oils, but we also use the word fat to refer to both fats and oils.

Fats do an excellent job carrying many flavours and making food tasty and satisfying. Fats enhance flavour, taste, aroma, crispness, juiciness, and tenderness. Fats also provide a smooth texture and a creamy feeling in the mouth. Eating a meal with fat makes people feel full because fat takes longer to digest. Fats in food are also crucial for the digestion and absorption of fat-soluble vitamins, vitamins A, D, E, and K.

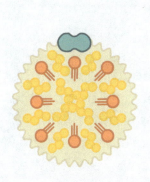 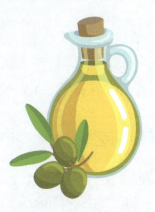 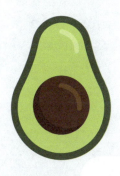

Fatty acids

Fatty acids are the basic components of lipids in plants and animals.

Fats we eat are broken down into triglycerides that travel in the blood to wherever they will be used or stored. Triglyceride is a fat molecule composed of one glycerol unit connected to three fatty acids. Over 90% of the fats in foods are in the form of triglycerides. Therefore, when we talk about fat in foods and the body, we talk about triglycerides. Naturally, most foods contain different types of fats: saturated and unsaturated fats (monosaturated and polyunsaturated fats).

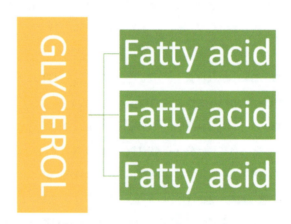

The illustration of a triglyceride

A saturated fatty acid has the maximum number of hydrogen atoms attached to every carbon atom. It is saturated with hydrogen atoms.

Unsaturated fatty acids have a double bond between the carbons in the middle of the molecule. If only one double bond exists, the fatty acids are called monounsaturated fatty acids (MUFA). If there are two or more double bonds in the fatty acids, the fatty acids are called polyunsaturated fatty acids(PUFA).

Fatty acids

Each type of fat in foods contains a mix of saturated, monounsaturated, and polyunsaturated fatty acids. However, one type of fatty acid usually dominates.

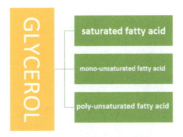

A possible structure of a fat

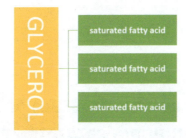

An illustration of a saturated fat

Saturated fat
The most significant sources of saturated fat in the North American diet are animal foods: cheese and pizza, beef, pork, poultry, butter, eggs, and so on. Animal fat often contains at least 50% saturated fat.

Most vegetable oils are rich in unsaturated fats, except tropical oils. Coconut oil, palm kernel oil, and palm oil are often called tropical oils, which are high in saturated fat. Tropical oils are used in processed foods, such as commercial baked goods and frozen, non-dairy toppings.

Monounsaturated fat.

In nutrition, monounsaturated fatty acids are also called monounsaturated fats, which are fatty acids that have one double bond in the fatty acid chain, with the remaining carbon atoms being saturated single-bonded.

Examples of monounsaturated oils include olive oil, canola oil, and safflower oil. These oils are used in cooking and salad dressings. Canola oil is also used to make margarine. Nuts and seeds are also good sources of monounsaturated fat.

The molecular structure of oleic acid, a monounsaturated acid.

It is the primary fatty acid in olive oil and canola oil

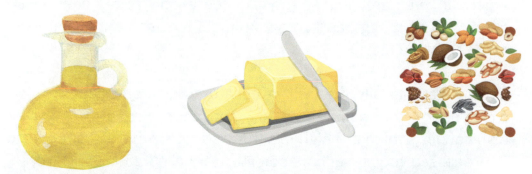

Polyunsaturated fat.

In nutrition, polyunsaturated fatty acids, also called polyunsaturated fats, are fatty acids that contain more than one double bond in their backbone. Polyunsaturated fats are fats in which the constituent hydrocarbon chain possesses two or more carbon–carbon double bonds. Polyunsaturated fat is primarily found in nuts, seeds, fish, seed oils, and oysters.

Polyunsaturated fats are found mainly in corn, soybean, and sunflower oils. These oils are commonly used in salad dressings, cooking oil, and baking. Nuts and seeds also contain polyunsaturated fats.

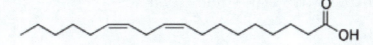

Chemical structure of the polyunsaturated fat, linoleic acid.

In summary, saturated fats are found primarily in animal foods such as meat and dairy. Monounsaturated and polyunsaturated fats are predominantly found in plant-based foods, such as vegetable oils, nuts and seeds.

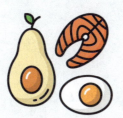
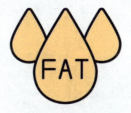

Essential fatty acids

What are essential fatty acids?

Essential fatty acids (EFA) are the fatty acids that can not be synthesized by the human body but are required by our body to maintain health. These must be ingested through diet.

The essential fatty acids are alpha-linolenic acid (ALA) and linoleic acid (LA).

Alpha-linolenic acid, also called ALA, is an omega-3 fatty acid.

Linoleic acid, also called LA, is an omega-6 fatty acid.

The body can make most of the fatty acids that it needs except for these two essential fatty acids.

Both of them are polyunsaturated acids. These essential fatty acids are vital to the health of your body cells and your healthy immune system. They are also needed for infants and children to grow and develop properly.

Alpha-Linolenic acid (ALA), an omega-3 fatty acid

Linoleic acid (LA), an omega-6 fatty acid

Essential fatty acids

Linoleic acid (LA) is categorized as an omega-6 fatty acid because its double bonds appear after the six carbons in their molecular chain from the omega end. Alpha-linolenic acid (ALA) is the leading omega-3 fatty acid found in food, and its double bonds appear after the 3rd carbon in the molecule chain from the omega end. Omega-3 fatty acids, along with omega-6 fatty acids, are heart-healthy.

Alpha-Linolenic acid (ALA), an omega-3 fatty acid

Linoleic acid (LA), an omega-6 fatty acid

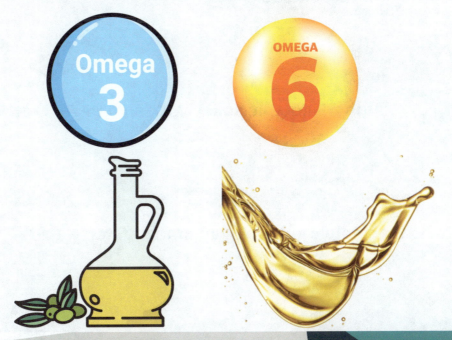

Food sources of essential fatty acids

Which foods contain linoleic acid or ALA?

Linoleic acid (LA), an omega-6 fatty acid, is found in vegetable oils such as soybean, corn, safflower, and sunflower.

Margarine, salad dressings, and mayonnaise all have omega-6 fatty acids.

Alpha-linolenic acid (ALA), an omega-3 fatty acid, is found in several oils, including canola, flaxseed, walnut, soybean, or margarine made with vegetable oils.

Ground flaxseed, walnuts, and soy products have omega-3 fatty acids.

Alpha-Linolenic acid (ALA), an omega-3 fatty acid

Linoleic acid (LA), an omega-6 fatty acid

DHA and EPA

Two other vital omega-3 fatty acids in our diets are DHA (docosahexaenoic acid) and EPA (eicosapentaenoic acid). These two fatty acids, DHA and EPA, are essential for heart and brain health, cognitive health, and eyes.

DHA and EPA are found primarily in fatty fish. Almost the only source of DHA and EPA is seafood, especially fatty fish such as salmon, mackerel, sardine, halibut, bluefish, trout, and tuna. Lean fish like haddock, cod, flounder, and sole contain only small amounts of DHA and EPA. DHA and EPA are not found in any plant foods. For children, eggs and milk are fortified (The process of enriching foods with nutrients) with DHA and EPA.

DHA is an essential nutrient for healthy eyes and brain as DHA is found in high concentrations in the retina of your eyes and your brain and is especially important for proper vision and brain development during pregnancy and infancy. In addition, DHA and EPA are excellent for heart health. They may help reduce blood pressure, clots, and triglyceride levels. DHA and EPA are also vital for cognitive health and are used to lessen symptoms in people with depression.

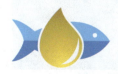

Cholesterol

Cholesterol, the fat maintaining cell integrity and functions

What is cholesterol?

Cholesterol is a substance that maintains cell integrity and functions. Cholesterol is made in the body and is present in every cell.

Cholesterol is also a member of the lipid family. Your body needs cholesterol to function normally. Cholesterol is part of every cell membrane and is present in every cell in the body. Cholesterol is present in brain and nervous system cells, muscles, skin, liver, and skeleton. Besides maintaining cell membranes, the body uses cholesterol to make the following essential substances to support the body's functions:

- Bile acids, which allow the digestion of fats;
- Many hormones. Hormones are chemical messengers in the body. Hormones enter the bloodstream and travel to a target organ to influence what the organ does, such as the sex hormones estrogen and testosterone;
- Vitamin D.

Because the body makes its cholesterol, cholesterol is not an essential nutrient.

Which foods contain cholesterol? Cholesterol is found only in animal foods. Eggs, meat, and whole milk provide most of the cholesterol we consume; these sources are also rich in saturated fat.

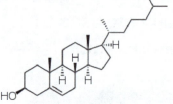

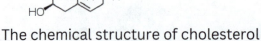
The chemical structure of cholesterol

Fats in the body

What do Fats do in the body?

Fat does lots of essential things in the body. And fat accounts for about 15%-30% or more of your weight, depending on the body's composition.
Fat is an essential nutrient for the human body; fat is part of all body cells. Fat plays the following crucial roles in the human body:

Fat is involved in the absorption and transport of the body's fat-soluble vitamins (A, D, E, and K).
Certain fat-containing foods provide the body with the essential fatty acids which the body can not make. The essential fatty acids for the human body are alpha-linolenic acid (an omega-3 fatty acid) and linoleic acid (an omega-6 fatty acid). The essential fatty acids are needed for body maintenance and are especially critical for the development and growth of children and infants. The essential fatty acids are important for healthy cells, and they play crucial roles in the proper functioning of the immune system.

Fats provide energy to us. One gram of fat yields nine calories, compared to 4 kcalories for one gram of carbohydrate or protein. Most cells store only tiny amounts of fat, but specific cells, called fat cells or adipose cells, can accumulate loads of fat. Your fat cells can increase while growing up and even during adulthood.

At least 50% of stored body fat is located under the skin, where fat provides insulation, optimum body temperature, and a cushion around critical organs by acting like shock absorbers.

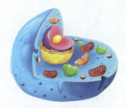
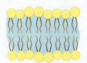

The digestion of fat in the body

Fat must first be digested and absorbed to perform its functions in the body. Fats are difficult for the body to digest and absorb because fat and water do not mix. Protein is soluble in water and will help the solubility of fats.

Fats are digested very little before they reach the upper part of the small intestine. Once fats reach the small intestine, the gallbladder is stimulated to release bile into the intestine. Bile contains bile acids that emulsify fat, meaning bile splits fats into small globules or pieces. This allows the enzyme to take off at least two fatty acids from each triglyceride so that they can be absorbed across the intestine wall.

Once absorbed into the cells of the small intestine, triglycerides are re-formed. The body wraps triglycerides and cholesterol in protein so they can float in the bloodstream. The resulting substance is called a lipoprotein. Lipoprotein is a combination of fat, protein, and cholesterol.

A lipoprotein called chylomicron carries mostly triglycerides from the intestine through the lymph to the blood and the body's cells. The cells either burn the triglycerides for energy or store them.

Proteins

Introduction

Proteins are macronutrients found in all living cells in animals and plants that play various important roles. The protein found in animals and plants is such an essential substance that the term protein derives from the Greek word "first."

Protein is contained in skin, hair, nails, muscles, and blood, to name just a few places. Proteins function broadly to build and maintain the human body, whereas carbohydrates and lipids are used primarily for energy.

Proteins, on the one hand, build the structure of the human body like Muscles, bones, hair, etc.; on the other hand, these perform many different functions, essential for the proper functioning of the body. We can break down proteins for energy if adequate carbohydrates are not available in the body.

Our body can manufacture proteins from amino acids. About half of the required types of amino acids can be synthesized in the human body, while the remaining types of amino acids must be obtained from the proteins in our foods.

After we eat protein, our bodies break it down into amino acids and use them for various processes, such as building muscle and regulating immune function.

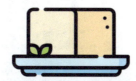

Protein in food

Proteins are macromolecules of amino acids linked together into a complex structure. Amino acids are the building blocks of proteins.

There are 20 different types of amino acids.

One of these 20 types, nine are essential amino acids, as they either can not be made in the body at all or can not be made in the quantities needed. You must get essential amino acids from food for your body to function normally.

The nine essential amino acids are histidine, leucine, isoleucine, lysine, methionine, phenylalanine, tryptophan, threonine, and valine.

The remaining eleven amino acids can be made in the body, called nonessential amino acids.

The eleven nonessential amino acids include alanine, arginine, asparagine, aspartic acid, cysteine, glutamic acid, glutamine, glycine, proline, serine, and tyrosine.

Protein is found in animal and plant foods. The amount of protein in food varies. Among plant foods, legumes, and nuts are excellent sources of protein. Animal foods like beef, chicken, and fish have more protein than plant foods. Most meats, poultry, and fish provide at least 20 grams of protein in a three-ounce serving.

Grains and vegetables provide some protein. For example, one slice of bread gives you about 4 grams of protein depending on the make and brand of the bread.

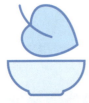 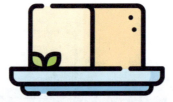

Nine Essential Amino Acids	Histidine
	Leucine
	Isoleucine
	Lysine
	Methionine
	Phenylalanine
	Tryptophan
	Threonine
	Valine

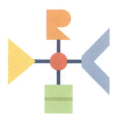
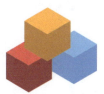

Non Essential Amino Acids 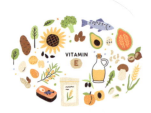	Alanine
	Arginine
	Asparagine
	Aspartic acid
	Cysteine
	Glutamic acid
	Glutamine
	Glycine
	Proline
	Serine
	Tyrosine

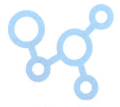
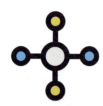

Protein | The macronutrient

Protein is a macronutrient and is a significant player in the diet. Protein is the body's building block forming and repairing muscles, skin, hair, and nails. Protein also enables many of the body's vital metabolic functions.

Proteins form the structure of tissues. They also carry molecules around the body to where they are needed. Proteins play important roles in biochemical reactions in the human body, including immune response and the production and deployment of hormones.

Proteins are made up of amino acids. Short chains of amino acids are called peptides, as amino acids connect with peptide bonds.

Longer chains of amino acids are called polypeptides or proteins. Protein chains can become complex as more and more chains join and fold in on themselves. The body breaks down protein chins into peptides to use for specific purposes as required. For example, the hormone insulin is a peptide.

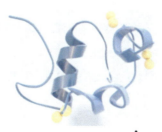

insulin

Insulin consists of two peptide chains, linked with two disulphide bridges shown in yellow

Complete and Incomplete Protein

The body can produce many amino acids to make peptides and proteins. However, nine amino acids are essential; they must be sourced from the diet as the human body can not make them. The nine essential amino acids are histidine, leucine, isoleucine, methionine, lysine, tryptophan, valine, threonine, and phenylalanine.

Humans do not synthesize these nine amino acids, which are dietarily essential or indispensable nutrients. These nine amino acids are called essential amino acids and are food sources of protein.

Food sources containing all nine essential amino acids in sufficient quantities are known as complete proteins. Complete proteins are found in animal products and a few plant sources.

Incomplete proteins are plant-based sources of proteins that do not contain all nine essential amino acids or do not contain sufficient amounts of essential amino acids to meet the body's daily requirements. Although "incomplete," they are no less valuable than complete proteins as protein needs are met throughout the day with meals and snacks.

Vegans and vegetarians are advised to eat a wide variety of protein-rich and fortified foods to ensure the consumption of all nine essential amino acids daily from complete and incomplete proteins.

The Twenty Amino Acids that make up proteins

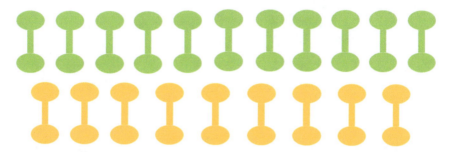

Nine Essential Amino acids

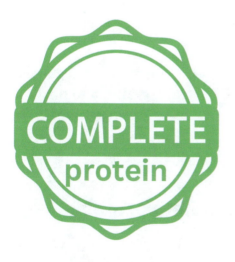

complete proteins contains all nine essential amino acids

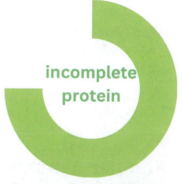

incomplete proteins contains fewer than nine essential amino acids

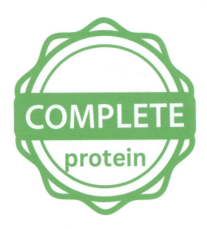

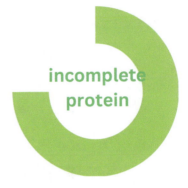

complete proteins contains all nine essential amino acids

incomplete proteins contains fewer than nine essential amino acids

animal-based protein: dairy products (milk, yogurt, and cheese), eggs, fish, and meat

plant-based protein soy and quinoa

nuts, seeds, legumes, grains, and many vegetables

Popular pairings of incomplete proteins
- lentils and rice
- oats and nuts
- brown rice and black beans
- hummus and bread or crackers
- lentils or beans with pasta

A complete protein, high-quality protein

Food proteins that provide all the essential amino acids in the proportions needed by the body are called high-quality proteins or complete proteins. Examples of complete proteins include animal proteins such as meat, poultry, fish, eggs, milk, and other dairy products.

Incomplete protein

Incomplete proteins are low in one or more essential amino acids. Plant proteins, including dried beans and peas, grains, vegetables, nuts, and seeds, are incomplete. The essential amino acid in the lowest concentration in protein is referred to as a limiting amino acid because it limits the protein's usefulness in the body.

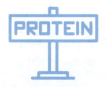
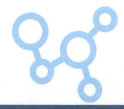

Complementary proteins

Although plant proteins are incomplete, it does not mean they are low quality. When certain plant foods, such as peanut butter and whole-wheat bread, are eaten over a day, the limiting amino acid in each of these proteins is supplied by the other food. Such combinations are called complementary proteins, and they yield complete protein.

This is the case when grains, such as whole grain bread, are consumed with legumes, such as peanut butter, or when rice (a grain) is eaten with beans (a legume). The combination of foods provides complementary proteins, yielding complete protein. For example, beans supply plenty of the essential amino acids lysine and isoleucine, both lacking in grains.

You also get complete protein by taking dairy with legumes, grains, nuts, and seeds. Some plant proteins, such as soybeans or quinoa, are complete proteins.

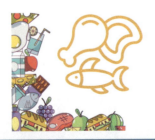
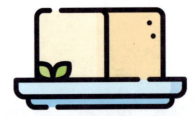

More about protein

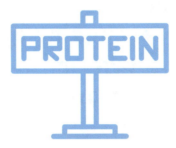

Protein comprises approximately 20% of the human body composition and is present in every cell. Protein is a Greek word for "of the utmost importance." Proteins are also called the workhorses of life because they provide the body with structure and perform various functions.

Protein is the major component of muscle. Protein is also required for proper immune system function, digestion, nail and hair growth, and many other body functions.

This chapter will discuss protein's roles within the body, how the body uses protein, and where to find healthy protein sources in our diet.

Protein in the body

Protein is an essential group of macronutrients required by our bodies. The functions of protein in our bodies are summarized as the following:

- Protein builds and maintains the body, and protein acts as a structural component of the body.
- Protein is a component of many enzymes, hormones, and antibodies.
- Protein helps transport iron, fats, minerals, and oxygen.
- Protein helps maintain fluid and acid-base balance.
- Protein helps blood clot when bleeding.
- Protein provides energy as a last resort. The body's primary energy source is carbohydrates and fat; protein is the last energy resort.

Protein in the body

The proteins we eat in food only become part of proteins in our bodies once they are broken down into single amino acid units during digestion and then used by our cells to make new proteins.

Protein digestion starts in the stomach when stomach acid uncoils the proteins enough to allow enzymes to enter them to do their work. An enzyme in the stomach begins splitting apart amino acids in proteins.

In the body, the instructions to make proteins reside in the cell's core, or nucleus, in each of your cells. The genetic material instructing the protein synthesis present in the nucleus of the cell is DNA. DNA is the abbreviation of deoxyribonucleic acid. Every human cell contains the same DNA, the master plan for cell function and reproduction. The exception is the mature red blood cells, which have no nucleus in them.

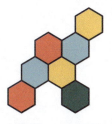
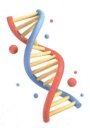

Protein in the body

Segments of each DNA molecule are called genes. A gene carries instructions that allow a cell to produce something, often a protein. There are thousands of genes in each of your cells with instructions to make many different proteins.

The supply of amino acids in the blood and the body's cells comprise the amino acid pool. Amino acids from foods and those from body proteins that have been disassembled stock this pool. Suppose your body makes a protein and can not find an essential amino acid. In that case, the protein production process can not be completed, and the uncompleted protein is degraded. In this manner, the human body recycles its proteins.

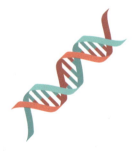
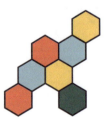

Protein in the body

Protein is part of most body structure: build and maintain the body; is part of many enzymes, hormones, and antibodies; transport substances around the body; maintain fluid and acid-base balance; can provide energy for the body; and helps in blood clotting.

Proteins function as part of the body's structure. Protein can be found in the skin, bones, muscles, hair, nails, blood vessels, digestive tract, and blood. Proteins also give structure to individual cells. Collagen, the most abundant protein in the body, is the major protein in bones, ligaments (which hold bones together), and tendons that attach muscles to bones. To a certain extent, collagen is the glue that keeps us together.

Proteins are used for building and maintaining body tissues. Worn-out cells are replaced throughout the body at regular time intervals. For instance, A skin cell lives only about one month. Skin is constantly being broken down and rebuilt, like most body cells. The cells that line the gastrointestinal tract are replaced every few days.

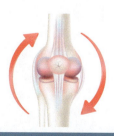 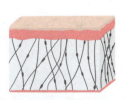 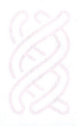

Enzymes, the proteins with specific biochemical roles

Enzymes are, in nature, proteins that perform some specific biochemical reactions. The enzyme's job is to provide a site for a biochemical reaction and lower the time and energy it takes for that biochemical reaction to take place. Hundreds of chemical reactions occur in cells every second, most requiring enzymes. Enzymes have specific sites where only particular substrates can fit into their active sites. Nearly all biochemical reactions require a specific enzyme. All bodily functions, including the breakdown and absorption of food in the stomach and small intestine, the transformation of nutrients into substances a cell can use, and the building of all macromolecules and proteins, require enzymes.

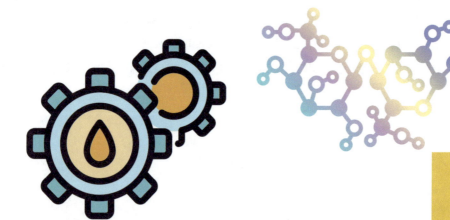

Proteins have roles in hormone synthesis.

Hormones are substances produced by the endocrine glands. Proteins are responsible for hormone synthesis. Many hormones are made from protein.

The hormone is produced from an endocrine gland when the endocrine gland is stimulated. The hormone is then released into the blood circulation to its target cell. In the target cell, the hormone conveys a signal to initiate a specific reaction or cellular process.

For example, insulin is a hormone secreted by the pancreas to regulate the level of blood glucose. After eating a meal, your blood glucose levels rise. The pancreas releases the hormone insulin in response to the increased blood glucose. Insulin tells body cells that glucose is available and to take up from the blood and either store it or use it for making energy or building other molecules and substances for the body's use.

Protein provides protection

The skin's dense network of collagen fibers provides skin with structure and support and serves as a barricade against harmful substances. The critical components of enzymes and antibodies are proteins. The immune system depends on enzymes and antibodies to attack and destroy harmful invaders like bacteria, viruses, and other toxic substances. One example is an enzyme called lysozyme, which is secreted in the saliva and destroys the cell walls of bacteria, causing them to rupture.

Specific proteins circulating in the blood can be directed to build a molecular knife that destroys the cellular membranes of the intruders. White blood cells secrete antibodies to look over carefully or inspect the entire circulatory system, locating and eliminating harmful bacteria and viruses. Antibodies also initiate other factors in the immune system to look for, identify, and destroy unwanted intruders.

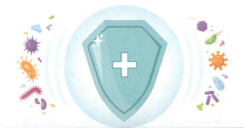

Protein for Structure and motion, the collagen

The most abundant structural protein in the human body is collagen, which makes up about 6% of total body weight and 30% of bone tissues. Collagen is a tough, fibrous protein in a highly ordered structure. Collagen comprises large proportions of tendons, ligaments, cartilage, skin, and muscle.

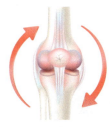 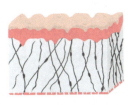

Collagen makes bones strong but flexible. The closely packed collagen fibrils in ligaments and tendons allow for synchronous mechanical movements of muscles and bones and the ability of these tissues to spring back after a move or action is complete. Collagen fibers in the skin's dermis provide structure, and the accompanying elastin protein fibrils give it flexibility. Collagen and elastin proteins secreted by the smooth-muscle cells surround blood vessels and provide structure and the capability of stretching back after blood is pumped through the blood vessels. Another structural fibrous protein is keratin. Keratin is what skin, hair, and nails are made of.

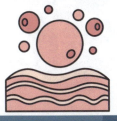 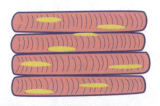

Proteins work to keep the fluid and Acid-Base Balance in the body

Proteins keep the acid-base balance and fluid balance in the body. Fluid balance refers to maintaining the balanced distribution of water in the body.

Water moves toward areas with higher concentrations of some solutes, such as glucose and proteins. To keep the water evenly distributed between blood and cells, proteins continuously circulate at relatively high concentrations in the blood.

The protein of abundance in the blood is the protein known as albumin. Albumin is a simple water-soluble protein, and its existence and presence in the blood make the protein concentration in the blood equal to that in cells. Thus, the fluid exchange between cells and the blood is balanced to preserve a dynamic state of equilibrium. Albumin functions as a buffer against abrupt changes in the concentrations of other molecules, thereby balancing blood acid-base balance and maintaining the steady state of equilibrium. The hemoglobin protein in the blood also keeps the acid-base balance by binding and releasing protons.

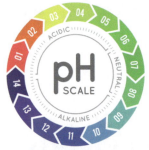
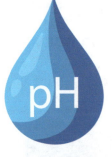

Protein in nutrients transport

Hemoglobin and albumin in the blood also play a role in substance transport. Albumin chemically binds to fatty acids, hormones, minerals, vitamins, and drugs and transports these substances throughout the circulatory system. Millions of hemoglobin molecules in every red blood cell bind oxygen in the lungs and transport oxygen to all the tissues in the body.

Many transport proteins are located in the cell membrane, helping get the required nutrients and molecules into the cell, as a cell's membrane is usually not permeable to large polar molecules. Some proteins are channels that allow particular molecules to move in and out of cells.

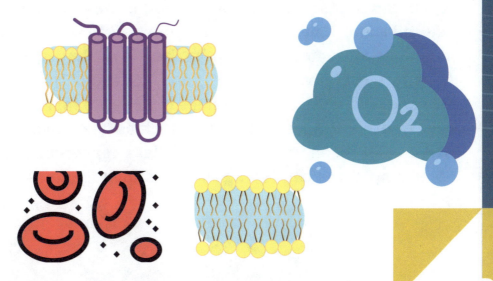

Protein's Roles in Wound Healing & Tissue Regeneration

Proteins have roles in all aspects of wound healing. Wound healing comprises three phases: 1) inflammatory phase, 2) proliferative phase, and 3) remodeling phase. For example, bleeding happens if there is a cut, and your flesh becomes inflamed and red.

After a few seconds, the bleeding stops; the healing process starts with proteins, which dilate blood vessels at the injury site. In the following proliferative phase, cells migrate and repair the injured tissue by installing newly made collagen fibers. The collagen fibers help pull the wound edges together. In the remodeling phase, more collagen is deposited, forming a scar. The wound healing process is markedly slowed if a diet lacks protein.

Tissue regeneration is ongoing in the body during healing. An exact functional and structural copy of the lost tissue will be regenerated in tissue regeneration. Tissue regeneration starts from the creation of new cells through cell division. Cell division requires different proteins, including enzymes, to synthesize RNA and proteins, transport proteins, hormones, and collagen. The cells of skin and hair, nails, and intestines regenerate rapidly. While cells of other tissues and organs, such as heart-muscle and nerve cells, regenerate at relatively less appreciable levels. For example, the cells lining the intestine regenerate every 3-5 days.

Energy Production

Some amino acids in proteins can be disassembled and used to produce energy. Approximately 10 percent of dietary proteins are catabolized daily to produce cellular energy. Suppose a person's diet does not contain enough carbohydrates and fats to serve as body energy. In that case, their bodies will have to use more amino acids to make energy, compromising the synthesis of new proteins and destroying muscle proteins. On the other hand, if a person intakes more protein than the body can use, the extra amino acids will be destroyed and transformed into fat.

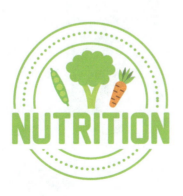
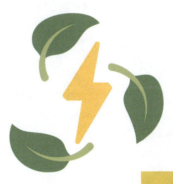

Phytochemicals & Phytonutrients

What are Phytochemicals, and what do they do?

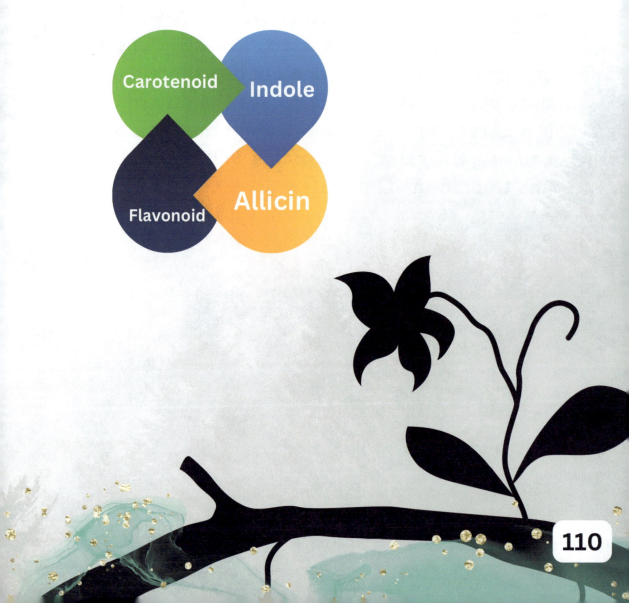

Phytochemicals & Phytonutrients

Phytochemicals are often referred to as phytonutrients, which are the nutrients found in plant-based foods such as fruits and vegetables.

Phytochemicals are naturally occurring compounds with potential health benefits. Phyto, from Greek, means plant. Phytochemicals are plant chemicals.

Unlike nutrients, phytochemicals or phytonutrients are not essential for life. Yet, because of their potential to promote good health, they have captured the attention of both academic research and the public.

Phytonutrients offer functional benefits beyond essential nutrition. Phytonutrients are substances produced by plants naturally to protect themselves against viruses, bacteria, fungi, insects, drought, and even sunlight. Additionally, phytonutrients provide the color, aroma, texture, and flavor that make many foods more appealing. For example, an orange has more than 170 different phytonutrients. Phytonutrients are concentrated in the skin or peel of vegetables and fruits.

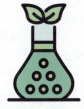

Phytonutrients

Phytonutrients are nutrients in plants that may provide some health benefits. Phytonutrients is a broader term that encompasses antioxidants. Phytonutrients include capsaicin, flavonoids, resveratrol, polyphenols, carotenoids, indoles, lignans, phytoestrogens, stanols, saponins, terpenes, anthocyanidins, phenolic acids, and many more. They are found in fruits and vegetables, grains, nuts and seeds, legumes, and some natural spices. Many phytonutrients act as antioxidants, but they have several other functions, such as inhibiting inflammatory responses, blocking the actions of specific enzymes, mimicking hormones, and altering cholesterol absorption.

Phytonutrients are present in small amounts in the food supply, and although thousands have been and are currently being scientifically studied, their health benefits remain largely unknown. Also largely unknown is their potential toxicity, which could be substantial if taken in large amounts as supplements. Moreover, phytonutrients often interact with each other as micronutrients such as vitamins and minerals. Therefore, eating various foods, including fruits, vegetables, and grain-baking foods, is recommended for a good balance of nutrients and phytonutrients.

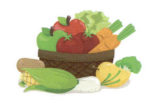

Phytochemicals/ Phytonutrients

In summary, the potential benefits of phytochemicals include the following:

- Reducing inflammation
- Strengthening the immune system
- Halting reproduction of damaged cells
- Preventing DNA damage and helping DNA repair
- Helping regulate hormones
- Helping prevent risks of cancer

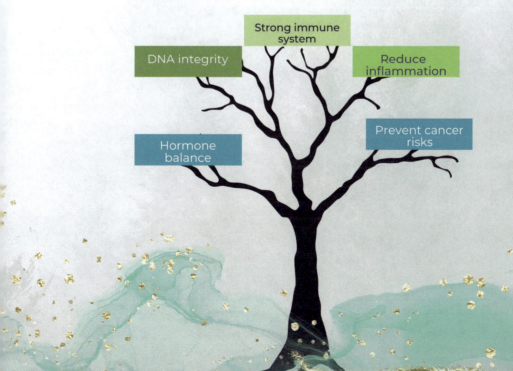

Phytochemicals categories

Phytonutrients are grouped according to their biochemical characteristics and similar protective functions in the human body. Most phytonutrients in vegetables and fruits fit into the following four groups: carotenoids, flavonoids, indoles, and allicin.

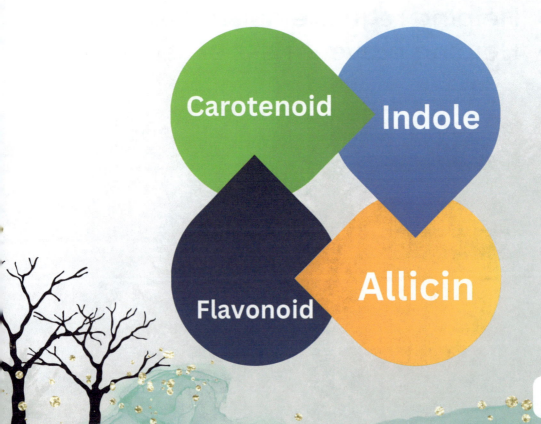

Carotenoids.

Carotenoids are fat-soluble phytonutrients.

Carotenoids are any class of highly unsaturated yellow to red-pigments occurring in nature. Nature's yellow, orange, and red colors come from over six hundred carotenoids. Carotenoids are also hidden by chlorophyll in some green plants.

The carotenoids such as beta-carotene, lutein, and lycopene are well-known substances in the fight to reduce the damage from free radicals. Beta-carotene supports and strengthens cellular antioxidant defenses by neutralizing free radicals that might damage cells. In addition, beta-carotene can be converted into vitamin A in the body. Beta-carotene is contained in yellow-orange vegetables such as carrots, pumpkins, sweet potatoes, apricots, cantaloupes, and papayas. Green vegetables like broccoli, kale, and spinach also have beta-carotene.

Another carotenoid is lycopene. Lycopene has antioxidative and anti-inflammatory functions and plays roles in immune modulation. Lycopene is contained in most red vegetables and fruits such as tomatoes, guava, pink grapefruit, and watermelon.

Other carotenoids important for maintaining eye health are lutein and zeaxanthin. These compounds exist in green vegetables such as asparagus, broccoli, Brussels sprouts, collard green, winter squash, kale, romaine lettuce, spinach, and Swiss chard. Corn, citrus fruits, kiwifruit, and egg yolks also have lutein and zeaxanthin.

lutein

lycopene

beta-carotene

zeaxanthin

Flavonoids

Flavonoids are water-soluble phytonutrients.

Flavonoids are any considerable class of plant pigments with a chemical structure based on or similar to flavone. Many biological effects of flavonoids are related to sending signals between cells.

Flavonoids also act as antioxidants and fight inflammation, possibly reducing the risks of heart disease. It may inhibit inflammation and tumor growth, aid immunity, and boost the production of detoxifying enzymes in the body.

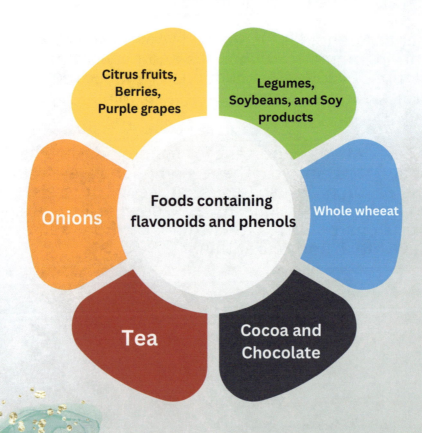

Indoles

Indoles are contained in cruciferous vegetables such as broccoli, cauliflowers, kale, cabbage, and Brussels sprouts.

Indoles may help detoxify carcinogens, limit cancer-related hormone production, block carcinogens, and prevent tumor growth.

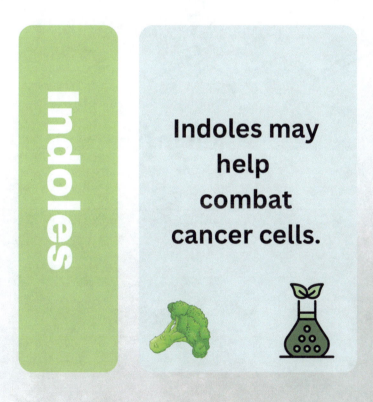

Allicin

Allicin is an organosulfur compound in garlic, chives, leeks, onions, and scallions.

Allicin may prevent cancer, lower cholesterol, and lower blood pressure. It may boost the immune system.

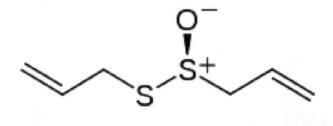

Allicin

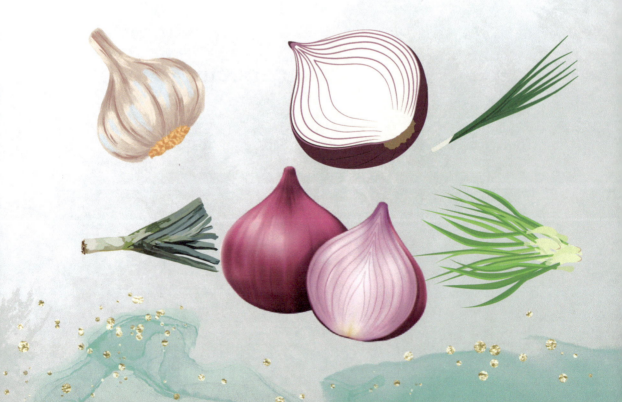

Phytochemicals, Selected Four classes of phytochemicals

Four classes of phytochemicals		
Phytochemicals	Foods	Health effects
Carotenoids	Yellow, orange, and red pigmented fruits and vegetables and some green vegetables. Some representative vegetables are carrots, pumpkins, winter squash, sweet potatoes, spinach, collard, kale, and bell peppers.	Carotenoids may reduce the risks of cancers, inhibit cancer cell growth, work as antioxidants, and improve immune response.
Flavonoids	<ul><li>**Black and green tea;**</li><li>**Cocoa and chocolate;**</li><li>**Onions;**</li><li>**Citrus fruits, berries, and purple grapes;**</li><li>**Whole wheat;**</li><li>**Legumes, soybeans, and soy products.**</li></ul>	They act as antioxidants and inhibit inflammation, possibly reducing the risks of heart disease. Flavonoids may aid immunity and boost the production of detoxifying enzymes in the body.
Indoles, Glucosinolates, sulforaphane	Cruciferous vegetables such as broccoli, cauliflowers, kale, cabbage, brussels sprouts	It may help detoxify carcinogens, limit the production of cancer-related hormones, block carcinogens, and prevent tumor growth.
Organosulfur compound, Allicin.	Allicin is an organosulfur compound in garlic, chives, leeks, onions, and scallion.	It may prevent cancer, lower cholesterol, and lower blood pressure. It may boost the immune system.

119

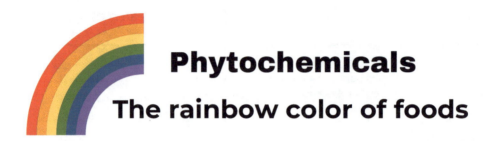

Phytochemicals
The rainbow color of foods

Phytochemicals Arranged in Color Groups

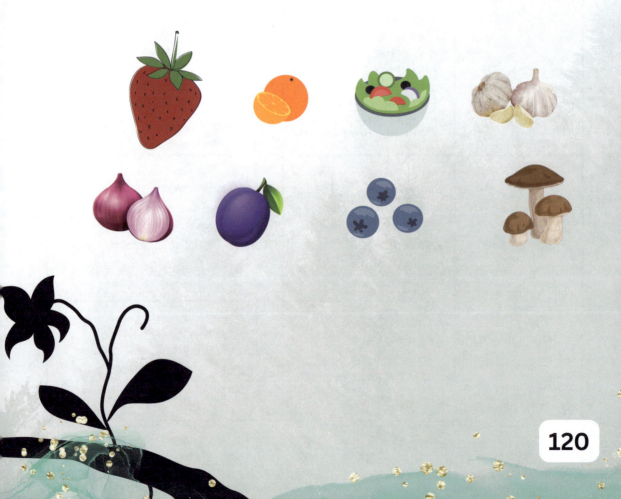

Phytochemicals

Next, we can group the phytonutrients according to the color they give foods.

Red color fruits and vegetables: The photopigment giving the red color is lycopene, which is a powerful carotenoid that may help maintain heart, vision, and immune health and may reduce cancer risks. When cooked, lycopene is more available to your body.

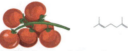

Orange and deep yellow: In these plant-based foods, carotenoids, flavonoids, and the antioxidant vitamin C may promote heart, vision, and immune health and reduce some cancer risks. The deeper the yellow/orange, the more carotenoids these foods have.

Green: The phytopigments of the color green are chlorophyll and lutein. In addition, the indoles also exist in green veggies and may help promote healthy vision.

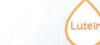

Purple and blue: The pigments giving purple and blue are anthocyanins, which provide a blue-purple color. Phenolics often are also contained in these foods, which may help with memory and urinary tract health and may help reduce cancer risks.

White and brown: The onion family contains allicin, which has anti-tumor properties. Allicin is found in onions, cauliflower, garlic, leeks, parsnips, daikon radish, mushrooms

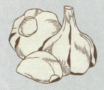 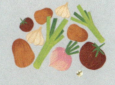

121

WHAT HAPPENS WHEN WE EAT?

The digestion, absorption of food, and metabolism

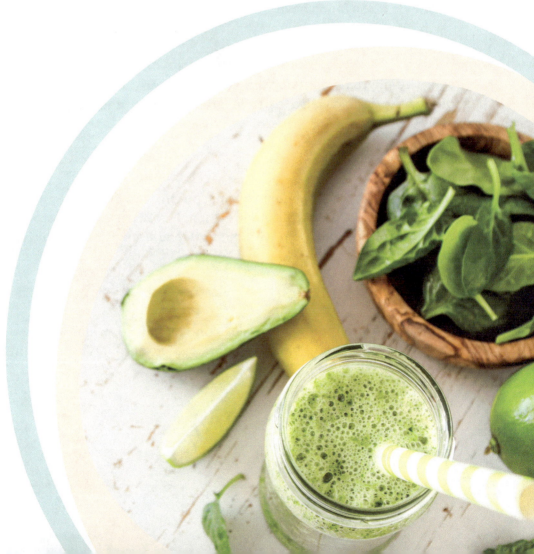

The digestion of food

To become part of the body, food must be digested and absorbed. Digestion is the process by which food is broken into its components in the mouth, stomach, and small intestine with the help of digestive enzymes and fluids. Enzymes are substances that speed up food's breaking down to help the body absorb the nutrients. Enzymes also perform other functions in the body.

Nutrients such as carbohydrates, fats, and proteins must be broken into components before they can be absorbed from the stomach or small intestines into the blood. Water, vitamins, and minerals need not be broken down further.

Before the body can use any nutrients present in food, the nutrients must pass through the walls of the stomach or intestines into the body's tissues; this process is called absorption.

Much digestion occurs in the small intestines, so nutrients such as carbohydrates, fats, and proteins can be absorbed. Nutrients are then transported in the blood through the body to the cells.

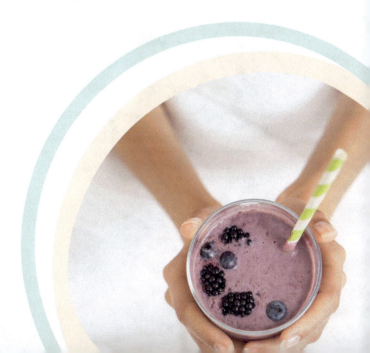

Metabolism

Metabolism refers to all the biochemical processes by which nutrients support life. Within each cell, metabolism takes place. Metabolism is divided into two parts: the building up of substances and the breaking down of substances.

Within each cell, nutrients such as glucose are split into smaller units to release energy. The energy is used to make heat to maintain body temperature or perform work within the cell. Substances such as proteins are built from their building blocks in every cell.

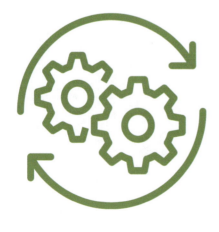
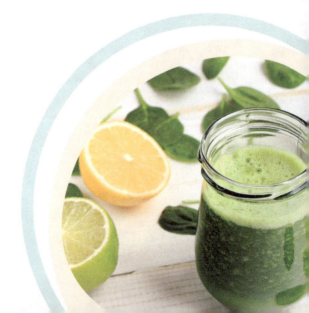

What happens when we eat, the food journey

Once we have eaten food, the food goes on a journey through the gastrointestinal tract, also called the GI tract or digestive tract. The gastrointestinal tract (GI) is a series of hollow organs joined in a long and twisting tube from the mouth to the anus. The hollow organs that comprise the GI tract are the mouth, pharynx, esophagus, stomach, small intestine, large intestine, rectum, and anus. The digestive system consists of the GI tract and solid organs like the liver, pancreas, and gallbladder. The ingested food is digested to extract nutrients and absorb energy, and the waste is expelled at the anus as feces. The gastrointestinal tract is so busy that the cells lining it are replaced every few days.

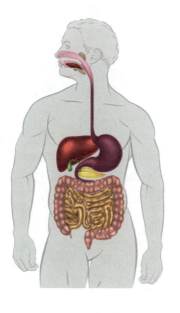

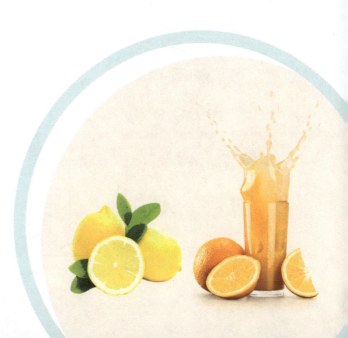

Digestion in Mouth- Formation of Bolus

The digestive system starts with the mouth. Your tongue and teeth help with chewing. It moves food around the mouth during chewing. Your teeth grind and break down food. Chewing is necessary because it breaks up the food into smaller pieces to be swallowed.

Saliva is a fluid secreted into the mouth from the salivary glands, contains important digestive enzymes, and lubricates the food so that it may pass readily down the esophagus. Digestive enzymes help break down food into forms of nutrients that the body can use. The tongue rolls the chewed food into a ball to be swallowed. This ball is called a bolus.

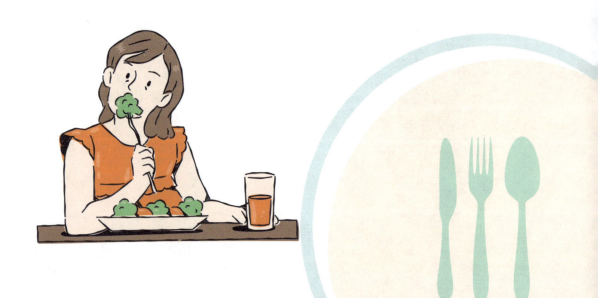

Digestion in Esophagus and Stomach- Formation of Chyme

When swallowed, food enters the pharynx and then the esophagus, a muscular tube about ten inches long that leads to the stomach. Food is propelled down the esophagus by peristalsis, the rhythmic contractions of muscles in the wall of the esophagus. Peristalsis also helps break up food into smaller particles. Food then passes from the esophagus into the stomach.

The stomach is a muscular sac that holds about four cups of food when full. The stomach makes an enzyme that helps in protein digestion and an acid that destroys harmful bacteria. The stomach has the strongest muscles and thickest walls of all the organs in the digestive tract. The food now has a semi-liquid consistency called chyme and is passed into the first part of the small intestine in small amounts. Liquids leave the stomach faster than solids, and carbohydrates and protein foods leave faster than fatty foods. The stomach absorbs few nutrients, but it does absorb alcohol. It takes 1.5 to 4 hours for the stomach to empty after eating.

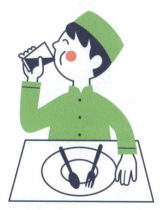
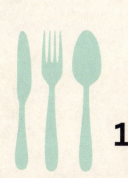

Digestion and absorption in Intestines

The small intestine receives the digested food from the stomach and enzymes from other organs, such as the pancreas. The small intestine produces digestive enzymes, and the liver makes bile to break down fat. Most digestion and absorption are completed in the first half of the small intestine. On the folds of the intestinal wall are tiny finger-like projections called villi. Nutrients are absorbed across the villi into the body, where they are transported to cells through the blood.

The large intestine also called the colon, is located between the small intestine and the rectum. One of the functions of the large intestine is to receive the waste products of digestion and pass them on to be eliminated. Waste products are materials that are not absorbed into the body. The large intestine absorbs water, some materials, and a few vitamins from bacteria residing there. Bacteria are normally found in the large intestine and are necessary for a healthy intestine. Intestinal bacteria make some important substances, such as vitamin K; they also can digest some components of foods, such as fiber. The rectum stores the waste products until they are released as solid feces through the anus, which opens to allow elimination.

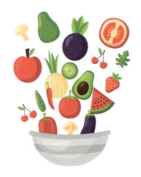

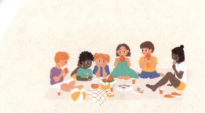

Balanced Diet

What is a Balanced Diet?

A balanced diet is one that meets the energy requirements of your body and provides the nutrients to keep it healthy. A balanced diet will have the following nutrients;
- Carbohydrates
- Healthy Fats
- Proteins
- Vitamins
- Minerals
- Water

In a balanced diet, Foods from all of the above groups are included in different proportions.

How to Choose Foods?

A handy way to remember how much of each food group to eat is the plate method. The USDA's "Choose My Plate" initiative recommends:
- Filling half your plate with fruits and vegetables
- Filling just over one-quarter with grains
- Filling just under one quarter with protein foods
- Adding dairy on the side (or a nondairy replacement)

People allergic to dairy products should go for nondairy products which provide similar nutrients.

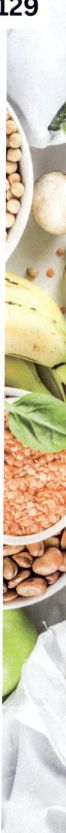

Antioxidants and free radicals

Natural Antioxidants from foods

Vitamins A, C, E, and the mineral selenium are the four significant antioxidants in our foods. In addition, other nutrients from plant-based foods, called phytonutrients, such as carotenoids, lipoic acid, and phenolic acids, also perform antioxidant functions guarding body cells against attacks by free radicals.

Vitamins A and E are essential vitamins required by our bodies, and they are also important antioxidants protecting cells from being damaged by free radicals. Vitamins A and E also help spare another antioxidant, glutathione. Glutathione can protect cellular components from damage caused by reactive oxygen species, such as free radicals, peroxides, lipid peroxides, and heavy metals. In addition, vitamin C and other phytonutrients such as carotenoids, lipoic acid, and phenolic acids all have antioxidant functions. The following table summarizes the significant antioxidants existing in our foods.

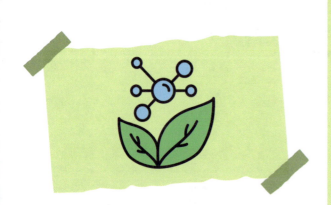
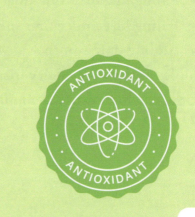

The Role of Antioxidants

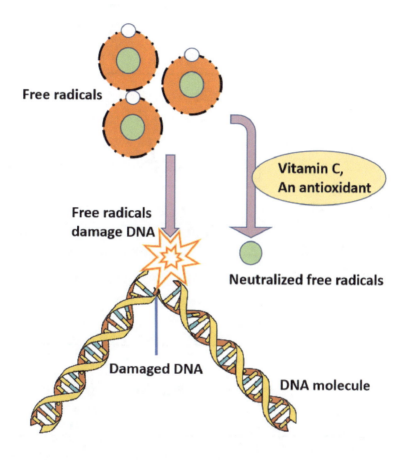

Antioxidants such as vitamin C can quench and neutralize free radicals and prevent them from attacking healthy cells and damaging the DNA in the cells.

A summary table of antioxidants

Antioxidant	Functions attributed to antioxidant capacity
Vitamin A	Protects cell membranes, prevents glutathione depletion, maintains free radical detoxifying enzyme systems, reduces inflammation
Vitamin E	Protects cellular membranes, prevents glutathione depletion
Vitamin C	Protects DNA, RNA, proteins, and lipids, aids in regenerating vitamin E
Carotenoids, a group of phytonutrient	Free radical scavengers
Lipoic acid, a phytonutrient	Free radical scavenger, aids in regeneration of vitamins C and vitamin E
Phenolic acids, a group of phytonutrients	Free radical scavengers protect cellular membranes.

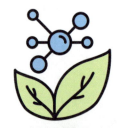
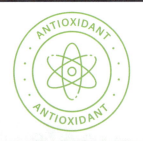

Free radicals, the oxidants in the human bodies

Free radicals are produced in our bodies when the foods we eat are converted to the energy we rely on. Factors from the environment can also trigger the generation of free radicals.

Energy sources and environmental substances can add to or accelerate the production of free radicals within the body. For example, exposure to excessive sunlight, smoke, heavy metals, ozone, asbestos, other toxic chemicals, and ionizing radiation increases the number of free radicals in the body. These factors trigger the formation of free radicals in the body.

Excessive exposure to environmental sources of free radicals can contribute to some related diseases by overwhelming the body's detoxifying systems to eliminate excess free radicals and repair the oxidative damage caused by free radicals.

Oxidative Stress caused by free radicals

Free radicals can cause oxidative Stress in the body. Oxidative Stress refers to an imbalance in any cell, tissue, or organ between the amount of free radicals and the capabilities of the detoxifying and repair systems in the body. Free radicals can attack body cells and tissues. However, our bodies can repair these damages when the number of free radicals is under reasonable control within the body's self-defense capabilities. On the other hand, if the free radical-induced damage is left unrepaired, the damage caused by free radical attacks can impair lipids, proteins, RNA, and DNA in cells, leading to inflammations and diseases.

The body's balanced defence, the two sides of free radicals

Free radicals have positive effects required by the body's immune system

While our bodies have acquired multiple defenses against free radicals, the human body also uses free radicals to support its functions. The immune system uses the cell-damaging properties of free radicals to kill pathogens. A pathogen is any disease-producing agent, especially a virus, bacterium, or other microorganism.

Free radicals can benefit the human body as they can kill pathogens. Free radicals are not always as harmful as attacking healthy body cells. However, they are also required by the immune system for the body's defense. Immune cells engulf an invading pathogen, such as bacteria; the pathogen is then exposed to free radicals, such as hydrogen peroxide, which destroys the pathogen. Scientific studies also suggest free radicals such as hydrogen peroxide can act as a signaling molecule that calls immune cells to injury sites and aid with tissue repair when the body gets cut.

Free radicals are necessary for many other bodily functions as well. For example, the thyroid gland synthesizes its free radical, hydrogen peroxide, which is required to synthesize thyroid hormone. In addition, reactive oxygen and reactive nitrogen species (free radicals containing nitrogen) interact with proteins in cells to produce signaling molecules. Some free radicals control their synthesis by acting as signaling molecules and regulating cell growth, development, reproduction, death, metabolism, and stress responses. Therefore, everything has two sides; we need a self-balancing body system.

Phytonutrients & Antixodants

Phytonutrients are nutrients in plants that may provide some health benefits. Phytonutrients is a broader term that encompasses antioxidants. Phytonutrients include capsaicin, flavonoids, resveratrol, polyphenols, carotenoids, indoles, lignans, phytoestrogens, stanols, saponins, terpenes, anthocyanidins, phenolic acids, and many more. They are found in fruits and vegetables, grains, nuts and seeds, legumes, and some natural spices. Many phytonutrients act as antioxidants, but they have several other functions, such as inhibiting inflammatory responses, blocking the actions of specific enzymes, mimicking hormones, and altering cholesterol absorption.

Phytonutrients are present in small amounts in the food supply, and although thousands have been and are currently being scientifically studied, their health benefits remain largely unknown. Also largely unknown is their potential toxicity, which could be substantial if taken in large amounts as supplements. Moreover, phytonutrients often interact with each other as micronutrients such as vitamins and minerals. Therefore, eating various foods, including fruits, vegetables, and grain-baking foods, is recommended for a good balance of nutrients and phytonutrients.

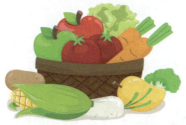

Units of Measurement

In this book, two systems of commonly used measurements are used: Metric and US customary.

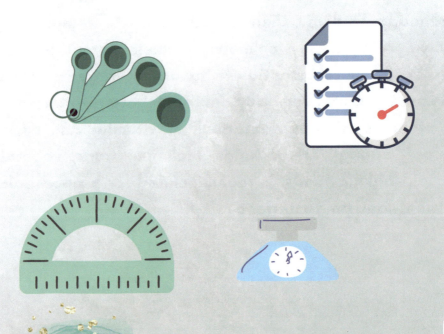

The commonly used prefixes for the Metric System

Prefix	meaning
Micro- (µ)	0.000001 (one millionth)
Milli- (m)	0.001 (one thousandth)
Centi (c)	0.01 (one hundredth)
Deci- (d)	0.1 (one tenth)
Kilo- (k)	1000 (one thousand times)

The Mass Units

Metric system	US customary system	Conversions
Microgram (µg)	Ounce (oz)	1 oz = 28.35 g
Milligram (mg)	Pound (lb)	1 lb = 16 oz
Gram (g)		1 lb = 454 g
Kilogram (kg)		1 Kg = 2.2 lbs

Interconversions between microgram, milligram and gram

Prefix	meaning
Microgram (abbreviated as mcg)	one microgram (mcg) = 0.000001 gram one mcg = 0.000001 gram
Milligram (abbreviated as mg)	one milligram (mg) = 0.001 gram one mg = 0.001 gram

  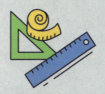

The Volume units

Metric system	US customary system	Conversions
Milliliter (mL)	Teaspoon (tsp)	1 tsp=5 ml
Deciliter (dL)	Tablespoon (tbsp)	1 tbsp = 3 tsp= 15 ml
Liter (L)	Fluid ounce (fl oz)	1 fluid oz= 2 tbsp = 30 ml
one liter = 10 deciliter (dL)	Cup (c)	1 cup= 8 fluid ounce = 237 ml
one liter= 1000 milliliter (mL)	Pint (pt)	1 pint = 2 cups = 16 fluid ounce
	Quart (qt)	1 quart = 4 cup= 32 fluid ounce = 0.95 L
	Gallon (gal)	1 gallon = 4 quart

The Length units

Metric system	US customary system	Conversions
Millimeter (mm)	Inch (in)	1 inch = 25.4 mm
Centimeter (cm)	Foot (ft)	1 foot = 30.5 cm
Meter (m)	Yard (yd)	1 yard = 0.9 meter
Kilometer (km)	Mile (mi)	1 mile = 1.6 kilometer

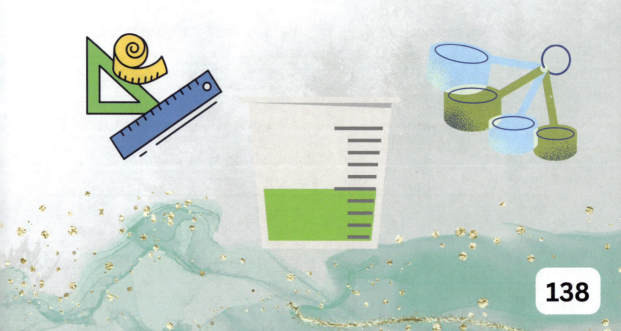

Thank you!

We thank you all for reading this book!
It is very nice meeting you, and thank you for being our readers and viewers.
We continuously strive to make high-quality content to provide informative food nutrition information and help make our lives healthier and happier.

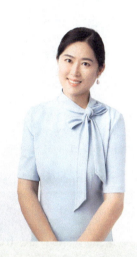

You can find our fun-to-watch videos for free on the following channels:

https://www.tiktok.com/@e.nutrition

https://www.youtube.com/@sutasty

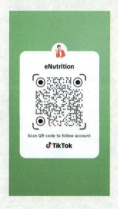

Again, it is very nice meeting you, and thank you for being our readers and viewers.
We continuously strive to make high-quality content to provide informative food nutrition information.

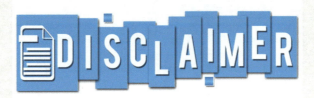

Disclaimer

This book is intended to provide broad guidance only and is not a substitute for professional medical advice, diagnosis, or treatment. If you have any concerns about your medical issues, dietary needs, or your interest in, questions about, or usage of dietary supplements, or what could possibly be best for your overall wellness, you must always seek the opinion of your physician or fellow licensed healthcare expert.

Never disregard or delay seeking professional medical advice based on a concept you read in this book, e-book, on our website, video & audio, articles or social media.

The author and publisher of this book are not medical professionals, and the information provided throughout is based on research, personal experience, and general health and wellness information and expertise. While every effort has been made to ensure the precision and accuracy of the information provided, the author and publisher render no implicit or explicit representations or assurances concerning the content contained in this book's completeness, accuracy, reliability, suitability, or availability for any purpose.

The reader acknowledges full responsibility for any actions taken in reliance on the information in this book. The author and publisher bear no responsibility for any direct, indirect, consequential, or incidental damages resulting from the use or inability to use the material in this book.

Before undertaking any new health or wellness program, making dietary changes, or commencing a new exercise regimen, it is critical to consult a licensed healthcare expert. Individual results may vary, and no assurances are offered concerning the outcomes or effects of following the advice or suggestions in this book.

The information provided in this book should not substitute any medical advice. Any reference to third-party websites or resources is provided for convenience only and does not indicate endorsement of the material, perspectives, or services offered by other websites.

By reading this book, you consent that you have carefully reviewed this disclaimer; and you agree to utilize the knowledge contained therein at your own discretion. Always prioritize your health and well-being by seeking tailored counsel and direction from a certified healthcare practitioner.

SuTasty Inc. owns and regulates all content copyright, and any replication of this channel's content without permission is prohibited.

INDEX

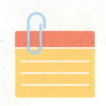

- Nutrients — **01**
- Disclaimer — **06**
- Water — **20**
- Carbohydrates — **27**
- Fats — **75**
- Proteins — **87**
- Phytonutrients — **110**
- What Happens When We Eat? — **122**
- Balanced Diet — **129**
- Antioxidants & Free radicals — **130**

About the author

The author of this book is Dr. Su Li, Ph.D.

Su has been in the food nutrition chemistry area for over twenty years. Su is a Canadian writer and video maker specializing in the food nutrition area.

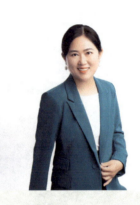

She has her food nutrition social media channels on YouTube, TikTok, and Facebook, where you can find high-quality, informative food nutrition videos for free. After years of creating food-nutrition-related videos, articles, and audios, she publishes books explaining the daily core nutrients: vitamins, minerals, and macronutrients (water, protein, fat, and carbohydrates) in a three-book series.

Su also explains the facts about antioxidants and phytonutrients in her books. Su transforms hard-understandable nutrition facts and information into easy-comprehensibly short articles for you to read.
You can find her and her fun-to-watch videos for free on the following channels:

https://www.tiktok.com/@e.nutrition
https://www.youtube.com/@sutasty

Again, it is very nice meeting you, and thank you for being our readers and viewers. We continuously strive to make high-quality content to provide informative food nutrition information and help make our lives healthier and happier.

Su's LinkedIn profile:
https://ca.linkedin.com/in/su9896

Made in the USA
Columbia, SC
29 June 2025

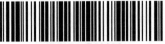